ALLENBY'S MILITARY MEDICINE

Life and Death in World War I Palestine

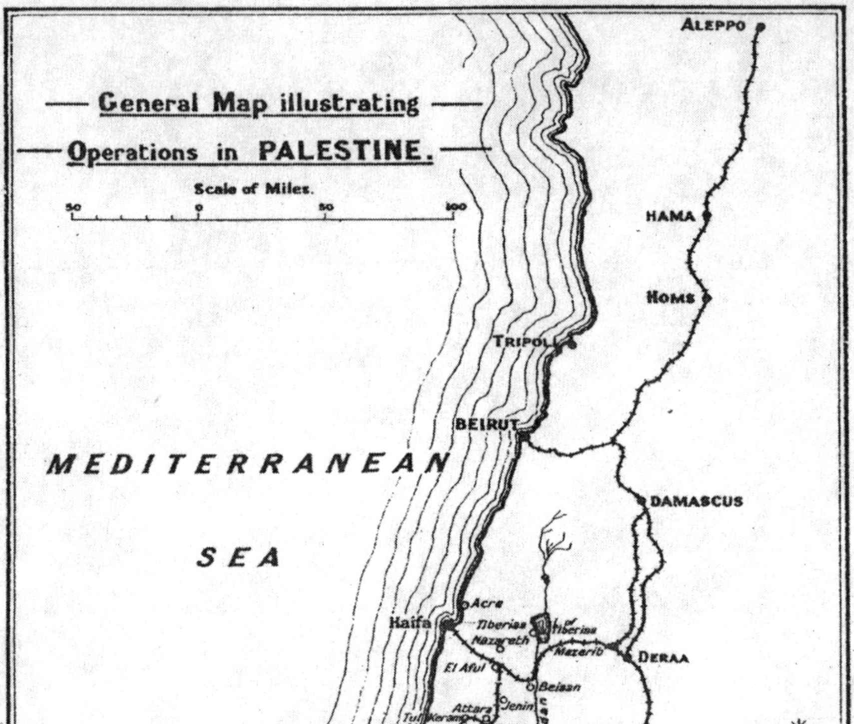

13. 2848 C. 5060/141. 1500.11.23.
H.M.S.O.,Cr.

ALLENBY'S MILITARY MEDICINE

Life and Death in World War I Palestine

ERAN DOLEV

I.B. TAURIS
LONDON · NEW YORK

Published in 2007 by I.B.Tauris & Co Ltd
6 Salem Road, London W2 4BU
175 Fifth Avenue, New York NY 10010
www.ibtauris.com

In the United States of America and Canada distributed by Palgrave Macmillan
a division of St. Martin's Press, 175 Fifth Avenue, New York NY 10010

International Library of Colonial History 6

ISBN: 978 1 84511 290 5

A full CIP record for this book is available from the British Library
A full CIP record is available from the Library of Congress

Library of Congress Catalog Card Number: available

Printed and bound by Thomson Press India Limited
From camera-ready copy edited and supplied by the author

Contents

FOREWORD

by

Major General Louis Lillywhite

MBE MSc MB BCh MFOM

This book is truly the result of a major piece of research, worthy of publication for the references alone. Although it has a medical theme, the story it tells has a much wider appeal. A glance at the Chapter headings indicates its relevance to those with a specific interest in General Allenby, and in military or medical history as well as to those with an interest in why things are as they are in the Middle East. However, the choice of anecdotes, the clarity of the descriptions, and the examination of the various participants also make it a book worthy of the attention of the casual reader. Eran Dolev guides the reader through the story in a manner that will hold the attention both of those without prior knowledge of the events described and those whose subject areas it covers.

In an illustrious and distinguished military career, the author has had two of the qualities that are so important in Medical Commanders, the ability to see issues from the perspective of the overall Military commander and the ability to balance the medical requirement with the realities of a military campaign. A Medical Commander has during the planning of an operation to on the one hand to fight to obtain the necessary resources and having obtained them to ensure that they are at the right place at the right time. However, the Medical Commander also has to take care that his demand for resources and priority is such that it does not compromise the outcome of a particular battle or campaign, for to do so may result in casualties being well cared for but the battle being lost, the military medical equivalent of "the operations was successful but the patient died". Nowhere do medical commanders face this dilemma more than in campaigns involving significant advances. This book contains many examples of where this dilemma occurred and Eran Dolev has managed to bring these dilemmas to life. Eran Dolev asks, I think rhetorically, in the final paragraph of the book whether the lessons are relevant to future wars. To those Commanders responsible for planning some of the campaigns of the late 20th and early 21st Century, the challenges faced, the issues arising, the arguments advanced, are all familiar. Indeed, the debate described in the book on the appropriateness or otherwise of forward surgical teams has continued unabated since their first use by the Australians under Allenby in 1917. The proponent and detractors of the argument on forward surgery in 1917 could almost have been present in person during the first and second Gulf Wars when the very same issue was debated with the very same emotion!

Allenby's campaign depended critically on logistic operations. Logistics is critical to success in most operations but is more so in desert operations when all that an Army needs for its survival has to be taken with it. Weaved in amongst the medical logistic challenges are described the approach to wider logistic planning and the achievements, such as building railway lines and pipelines behind the advancing Army, would bring credit on any modern day General. But planning is one thing and execution is another. It seems that Allenby was blessed by subordinate commanders who for the most part could understand their orders, were prepared to find ways to implement them, could respond appropriately when things went wrong and were able to improvise when faced with the unexpected. Again, many of the problems, such as blocked evacuation routes or medical units not where they were expected to be, would be recognised by modern day practitioners, even the unexpected (which to those with an interest in military history would not perhaps have been unexpected). In this category are the medical problems faced by Allenby's forces as they occupied civilian areas or came across demoralised or abandoned enemy inured that were faced, for example, by British Forces after the battle for Basra in the Second Gulf War.

Allenby's campaign was fought at a time when we were not as in control of infectious diseases as we are now, and thus some of the challenges that he faced are not as familiar to us. There are however similarities. The argument over whether any preventive medicine should be taken to minimise malaria has merely been replaced by arguments over which medication should be taken and it might be that the problems faced at the end of the campaign as a result of the influenza pandemic of that time are soon to be faced by today's Commanders.

Campaigns are of course rarely isolated affairs and are usually part of wider geopolitical events and the campaign in Palestine was no different. At its commencement the campaign was very much a backwater, overshadowed by the battles in Europe and by the defeat in the Dardenelles and with an enemy who seemed to be content with simply maintaining the Status quo. We gain an insight from the book at how a combination of initial success by a local commander prepared to take the initiative and local politics interacted to raise the global profile of the Theatre of operations, in turn leading to additional national resources being put into the campaign. In so doing the campaign led directly to the British mandate in Palestine which in due course led to the current political boundaries in that part of the Middle East. As one reaches the end of the book, one is prompted to ask oneself the question "If Allenby had not triumphed, and had not completely defeated the Turkish Armies and taken Jerusalem, would there today be an Israeli State?" Eran Dolev has dissected a campaign whose success depended in large part on the medical contribution, and which arguably led in due course to the existence of Israel.

The book is set in an area of historic and contemporary interest, addresses medical issues that remain relevant today, describes an outstanding leader winning a major victory, and brings it all alive with carefully selected anecdotes. This then is a book worth reading.

PREFACE

I was born in the city of Tel Aviv, Israel, then Palestine under the British Mandate. One of the main streets of my home town was Allenby Street. As a child I often wondered who was this foreigner after whom the street had been named. The more I learned about the period of the Great War in the Middle East and the man himself, the more I became fascinated by the subject in general and with Allenby in particular. Already as a youngster I could visit various places which had been important battlefields during the Palestine campaigns.

I now jump forward to the Six Days War in June 1967. The mission of our Airborne brigade was to participate in the capture of the town of Gaza and continue into the Sinai Desert. I served as the medical officer of the brigade and had to plan the medical treatment and evacuation of our expected casualties and later to execute the plan on the actual battlefield.

This was the first time I was exposed to the military tradition connected with the town of Gaza. I quickly became familiar with names of hills and strongholds in the area, as well as with various locations in the town itself. After the war was over, I was not surprised to learn that the very places which were so crucial for us in our battle of Gaza had been the key posts for the British forces during the three battles of Gaza fought in 1917. I served long periods of time in the Sinai Peninsula, the terrestrial bridge between Asia and Africa in times of peace and war, and became aware of the special problems this arid zone had created for so many generals throughout history.

Studying the various aspects of the Palestine campaign, I realized that though many memoirs and research works had been dedicated to this campaign, the issue of military medicine had not been studied in depth. I felt that studying this subject was not just my own obsession. I learned that the campaign in Palestine was unique among the various campaigns of the Great War. It was a mobile one, totally different from the trench war waged on the Western Front. It was also unique among the "side shows" of the Near East: the British thrusts at the Gallipoli Peninsula and in Mesopotamia were failures, while the campaign in Palestine was a success. But the unique feature of this campaign seemed to me to lie in the area of the exceptional relations between line officers and medical officers at all levels, inspired by the C-I-C.

When I retired from military service in 1983, after serving as Surgeon General of the Israel Defence Forces during the Lebanon War, and returned to my clinical and academic work, I could devote more and more time to an in-depth study of this subject. This book is the outcome of that research.

General Allenby, the successful commander of the Egyptian Expeditionary Force (EEF), was unique among the British generals during the Great War in his deep understanding of the importance of military medicine. The various EEF medical units functioned at the highest professional level throughout the whole Palestine campaign. It is a pity that most of the medical lessons attained during the Palestine campaign have been forgotten in the course of time.

Thus, as an Israeli citizen and as a physician and retired medical officer, I am very proud that almost sixty years after the British Mandate came to end, one can still find an "Allenby Street" in all our major cities.

The story of military medicine, an essential component of any campaign, is quite a complex one. It is not just a tale "of guns, and drums, and wounds" (William Shakespeare, *Henry IV*, Pt. I, Act I, Sc. 3).

Eran Dolev

ACKNOWLEDGEMENTS

I want to express my special thanks to two dear friends and distinguished scholars who read the manuscript, made many comments, found mistakes, and helped me clear up matters and avoid errors: Colonel (Ret.) Professor Robert J.T. Joy, the former Head and Chairman of the Department of Medical History at the Uniformed Services University of the Health Sciences (USUHS), Bethesda, Maryland, U.S.A., and Israel Defence Forces Colonel (Ret.) Yigal Sheffy, Ph.D., Tel Aviv University, Israel. I am very grateful to them both.

I wish to acknowledge the help of Nili and Amos Oz in Israel, Mrs. Deborah Owen in the U.K., and Mrs. Sara Lahat in both Israel and New York City. I also want to thank various friends too numerous to list here, who encouraged me at times when I considered my work a "mission impossible."

My sincerest thanks to Mr Yohai Goell, the Israeli editor who handled the book in the most professional manner. I wish to acknowledge his skill, dedication, and devotion. I acknowledge with gratitude the efforts of Mr Eli Oren, the Israeli producer of the book, who has demonstrated to me in the best possible way what is true professionalism .

Throughout the last twenty years I have discussed many topics in military medicine with my friend and distinguished colleague Major General Louis Lillywhite, MBE Msc Mb BCh MFOM, a truly experienced and knowledgeable Medical Officer. I am both honoured and privileged that he has written the foreword for this book

I am very grateful to the staff of the Liddell Hart Centre for Military

Archives at King's College, University of London; to the staff of the Department of Documents and the Reading Room, the Imperial War Museum, London; the staff of The National Archives (then the Public Records Office [P.R.O.]), at Kew, and the staff of the Wellcome Institute for the History of Medicine, London. There is no doubt in my mind that without the cooperation and full assistance of all these people, the task I took upon myself would have been much more difficult, if not entirely impossible. I would also like to acknowledge the positive attitude of the Rector of Tel Aviv University, which contributed towards the publication of this book.

Though all illustrative materials – photographs and maps – reproduced in the volume were published more than seventy years ago, I did attempt to trace the holders of copyright for the various photographs. Though the attempts proved unsuccessful, I wish to acknowledge the sources. Several photographs were published in 1918 by Cassell & Co., Ltd. of London, and I thank Cassell PLC, a division of The Orion Publishing Group, London. The maps and several photographs were published by HMSO, London, more than eighty years ago. HMSO rights are protected by Crown copyright for fifty years. I wish to acknowledge the source of these maps.

My thanks to my colleagues at I.B.Tauris for their full cooperation. It all began with Iradj Bagherzade, Ph.D., who was impressed by the material he had seen and initiated the process that ended in acceptance of the manuscript for publication by his publishing house. Wonderful cooperation continued with my editor in London, Ms Elizabeth Friend-Smith, who has always been there for me, and with Ms Kelly Hallett, the project manager, who has responded to several challenges that cropped up along the path towards production.

I dedicate this book to my wife Dalia for her patience, support, and assistance.

Eran Dolev

PROLOGUE

> 'War is a strange thing. On the one side you have all the signs of excessive hate and unbridled passion that show the innate madness that still lurks in the human soul. On the other hand you have all the signs of unselfish devotion and kindliness of spirit, even towards the man whom you have just struck in your hate, that show that there is, somewhere, a reserve of saving grace that rescues mankind from utter degradation.'
>
> A letter from Gallipoli dated 13 July 1915. Serjeant-Major R.A.M.C. WIHM, RAMC 1452, 11.

The Palestine campaign of 1917–1918 is considered one of the most successful fought during the Great War. No doubt it is among the most famous campaigns in modern times. It was won by the cavalry, which fought in the traditional manner, and led to the destruction of the Ottoman army. It also bore many historical and religious associations: the taking of Jerusalem, the Holy City, and a final battle that took place at Megiddo (biblical Armageddon). Many have compared the Palestine campaign to a crusade, ignoring the heterogeneous ethnic composition of the British army fighting in Palestine, which included many Muslim troops.

The Palestine campaign is remembered in the collective memory as a relatively pleasant experience. When compared to the Western Front, where high numbers of casualties were again and again mutually inflicted on the opposing forces, including casualties resulting from the use of gas shells, this campaign has been perceived as a positive experience. It was also the most successful campaign fought by British troops outside the Western Front.

Yet, from the beginning of the War until the Armistice, the British forces suffered 554,828 casualties during operations in Egypt and Palestine. More than 16,000 troops lost their lives: some 10,000 of them were either killed in action or later died of their wounds. The rest died from various diseases, primarily malaria. More than 50,000 soldiers were wounded on the battlefields and evacuated for treatment by various medical units, while about half a million were evacuated and treated for diverse diseases.[1] Thus, Field Marshal Michael Carver was right when he wrote that 'casualties were high in all three campaigns [against the Ottoman Army] both in action and from disease, and the sufferings of the soldiers in some respects were starker than on the Western Front.'[2] This was true not only in the Dardanelles and Mesopotamia, where the battles were eventually decided by disease, but also to some extent in Palestine.

The Palestine campaign of 1917–1918 was indeed unique in its medical aspects: it was not a medical disaster, as were most of the other campaigns fought outside the Western Front. This may explain why the medical features of this chapter in military history have not been thoroughly investigated and evaluated. One might find it quite amazing that whereas the medical aspects of the Gallipoli and Mesopotamian campaigns have been described and discussed in detail, the issue of military medicine during the Palestine campaigns has not received any real attention. Most probably the explanation lies in human nature: people tend to take great interest in extreme events and extraordinary people. Thus, historians tend to write about blunders and heroes. In this respect, the medical history of the Palestine campaign, where most of the operations were executed according to plan, seemed quite unattractive. The fact that the medical services performed most successfully during these campaigns did not seem too impressive.

One of the unique features of the Palestine campaign was the full cooperation received by the medical services from the commanding and staff officers at all levels and all times. This was an exception during the Great War, enhancing the status of the medical personnel in Palestine and allowing them to achieve more than on other fronts, where relations were quite different. No doubt this situation was inspired by the C-in-C, General Edmund Allenby, who considered the health of his troops to be a crucial issue.

The story of military medicine during the Palestine campaign of 1917–1918 is essentially a narrative of human suffering and agony as well as one of utmost devotion and successful medical and surgical work on the battlefields of the Middle East, far away from Europe.

1

MILITARY MEDICINE DURING THE GREAT WAR

'The whole object of the medical service in war is to provide men for the fighting line, to keep them fit, and, if sick or wounded, to make them fit and ready for further fighting as soon as possible.'

T.H. Goodwin, 'The Collection and Evacuation of Sick and Wounded from Front to Base,' *Military Surgeon* 40 (1917): 610.

British military medicine during the Great War was the outcome of a process of evolution and development in two different domains. The first reflected developments in various disciplines within the medical profession itself, mainly surgery and prevention of disease. The second was the outcome of military science and organization. Changes in strategic thought, tactical approaches, the efficiency and lethality of weapons, and the mobility of military units were but the main issues which to a large extent influenced military medical practice.

Modern military medicine is a defined field among the health professions that is concerned with the health of the troops. In contrast to civilian medicine, where professional obligations are restricted to the patients and to society, military medicine has a basic obligation to the military organization and to its missions. It includes the application of health science and medical practice in preventing disease among the troops as well as participation in the planning of operations. At the tactical level this enables better execution of missions by the supported unit. Military medicine includes the technical competencies of prevention, education, treatment, and organization. One of the hallmarks of military medicine as manifested by the military-medical personnel is total commitment and devotion to the unit, its people, and its mission.[1]

The practical meaning of modern military medicine on the battlefield has been the creation of the chain of medical responsibility: the professional organization which takes care of every battle casualty from the minute he is wounded through the various medical echelons, until convalescence.[2]

The first and constant link in the chain of medical care and evacuation, during various modern wars, has been the battalion or regimental Medical Officer (MO):

> The battalion MO is the most important individual in the medical organization. The duty of medicine in army is to enable the army to keep in health, to fight and win battles, and this duty is mainly accomplished through the battalion MO's. What is successful army sanitation but the sum of the apparently inglorious work of the battalion MO's? It is they who keep armies on their feet and preserve their health so as to maintain their activities in battlefield.[3]

When the battalion was engaged in active combat, its Medical Officer's task was to establish a Regimental Aid Post (RAP) in the rear of his battalion. The RAP was located as close to the firing line as possible, at a sheltered position when feasible, usually in a dugout, its distance from the firing line being about half a mile or less.[4]

The Medical Officer had under his command two medical orderlies and sixteen stretcher bearers, who were gathered from the battalion itself, with eight stretchers. This number could be increased according to needs. The bearers carried battle casualties from the firing line to the RAP. There casualties received first aid, were given to drink, and prepared for further evacuation to the next medical echelon. The MO was also in command of sanitary orderlies and was responsible for water purification in his unit.[5]

During combat, the MO would place himself not far from the Battalion Commander.[6] By this method, everyone knew where he was located and he himself was quite near to the main source of information. While in defence the RAP was located near the main communication trench which usually ran towards the rear.

The MO was expected to be with his battalion at all times. He would always try to be in touch with the next medical echelon, whose task was to clear casualties from the RAP after being attended by the MO. This enabled the MO and his team to continue to advance with his battalion.

Being a battalion MO was a very demanding task and one calling for great endurance. While serving at the front doctors were exposed to danger. Many of them lost their lives or were injured while attending casualties under fire. Utmost devotion and dedication were the hallmark of the Medical Officers' work everywhere. While all MOs fully identified with their task, there could be several levels of identification with the military organization: some doctors, when faced with extreme situations on the battlefield, took command of their units and behaved like line officers for a certain time. Others adhered to the Code of the Geneva Convention and did not carry weapons.[7]

While the MO was the first, the constant, and the crucial link in the chain of medical responsibility on the battlefield, the organization of British military medicine as a whole saw changes and developments during several military conflicts. The origins of British military medicine during the First World War might be sought in the South African Boer War (1899–1902) and its lessons. That was the first military conflict in which the Royal Army Medical Corps (RAMC), which had been established in 1898, took part. For British doctors, it was also the first 'modern war' in which prevention of wound infection by applying the attitudes of asepsis and antisepsis were emphasized at the various battlefields and at field hospitals.[8] During the war in South Africa, the evacuation of British casualties from the battlefield was organized along medical units, organized in echelons. Treatment of these casualties became integrated with the process of medical evacuation.

Though the concept of an integrated process of medical evacuation was clear to the RAMC, it was not efficient enough. During the Boer War, battle casualties were collected from the front line by stretcher-bearers who were organized in Bearer Companies. They further evacuated the casualties to the nearest Field Hospital, sometimes located far away from the combat zone. In many cases the work of these two separate bodies was not coordinated.

> Experience in the late war had shown that separate Bearer Companies and Field Hospitals distributed work unequally and wastefully. Too often the Bearer Company was unemployed, the Field Hospital overwhelmed. Combining the two, as had been tried by the volunteers, the Australians, and the Indian

> medical units, working alongside the RAMC, showed no such drawbacks. There was no duplication of control. Experience had also shown the need for divisibility of field units into functional sub-units with holding points – i.e. beds, and for a much larger proportion of stretchers and stretcher bearers.[9]

The outcome of this situation was the establishment of a new medical unit in the field: the 'field ambulance.' Replacement of the Bearer Company and the Field Hospital by the field ambulance took place in 1905. The main task of the new integrated medical unit was to free the combat units, namely their RAPs, from responsibility for retaining or evacuating their casualties, and it was structured accordingly.

The field ambulance was a medical unit commanded by a Lt-Col. RAMC. It included 10 officers and 224 other ranks, 165 of them being RAMC personnel while the rest were of the Royal Army Service Corps (RASC). The personnel of the field ambulance did not carry weapons. It was organized in three similar sections: 'A' Section, which included also the field ambulance's HQ, 'B,' and 'C.' Each of these consisted of two subdivisions: a stretcher-bearer subdivision whose task it was to collect and evacuate battle casualties from the RAPs, and a tent subdivision in which the patients, wounded or sick, were treated. Every stretcher-bearer subdivision included thirty-six bearers organized in nine squads.

The field ambulance was equipped with ten horse ambulance wagons, as well as general purpose wagons and carts, drawn by sixty-six horses, most of them draught and pack horses. During the Great War, ten motor ambulance cars were added to every field ambulance, increasing significantly its ability and the efficiency of medical evacuation.

The tent sub-division could accommodate 150 patients. Three field ambulances were allotted to every infantry division, and one to every Army Corps. Though field ambulances were divisional units, a field ambulance was usually attached to each brigade in a division. Field ambulance commanders received their professional orders from the divisional Medical Officer (the ADMS).[10]

According to the modus operandi of the field ambulance, casualties from the Regimental Aid Posts were collected by its stretcher-bearers after they had been attended by the regimental or battalion MO. The bearers evacuated these casualties towards the rear, either to the Advanced Dressing Station

(ADS) established by the field ambulance, or to the nearest point to which the horse-drawn or motor-driven ambulances could approach. From the ADS the bearers were expected to return immediately to the RAP in order to collect and evacuate more battle casualties.

During the early stages of the Great War on the Western Front, it was realized that the evacuation process was of itself an important factor in producing shock. The military doctors' conclusion was that evacuation of wounded soldiers should be as short and as convenient for them as possible. It was also found that early immobilization of broken limbs diminished further damage to the surrounding soft tissues and reduced the occurrence of shock. The use of the Thomas' splint at advanced medical units, for immobilization of fractured femurs, led to a reduction of the mortality rate of more than 30 percent among these cases. From 1916 on, the Thomas' splint was used at the field ambulance level.[11]

The ADS was established by the field ambulance about half a mile to one mile behind the battalions' RAPs for the brigade to which it was attached. Though better equipped than the RAP and more sheltered from enemy fire, it provided only limited medical treatment, mainly wound dressing and stabilization of fractured limbs. Emergency procedures were carried out at the ADS only when these were absolutely indicated. Casualties were evacuated from the ADS to the MDS (Main Dressing Station). One field ambulance could establish more than one ADS per brigade according to the situation on the battlefield.[12]

The MDS was established by the field ambulances for a division. It was usually formed by the 'A' (Headquarters) Section of a field ambulance. When several divisions operated on a narrow front, a Corps MDS was formed. In such a case, the Corps MDS was reinforced by personnel from field ambulances of other divisions. Conditions at the MDS were more comfortable for the patients, as well as for the surgical and medical teams. It was located relatively far away from the firing line (about a mile behind the ADS), being thus a much safer medical installation. This allowed the surgeons to operate on some of the casualties at the station, as well as to keep others for quite a long time. In some cases, the MDS might be replaced by a Casualty Clearing Station (CCS). All this meant, at least on the Western Front, that the MDS was usually established in a building and near a railway line.[13]

The MDS could accommodate and treat 400–500 casualties. It included subdivisions for 'Receiving' and 'Recording.' It was able to function as a

'Collecting Station' or a 'Dressing Station.' A Collecting Station was 'the place where slightly wounded men, able to walk, are collected, fed and rested before evacuation or return to their units.' A Dressing Station was 'the centre behind the lines to which wounded are sent from the RAP's to have immediate surgical or medical treatment before being carried or directed to the CCS.'[14]

The term 'Receiving Station' or 'Divisional Receiving Station' was used to describe a medical detachment of the field ambulance which was located near a railhead. It was the last medical echelon at the divisional level and usually was formed by the immobile section of an ambulance.[15] In special cases, where a whole corps was fighting in the same arena, the three immobile sections of each division were amalgamated into one unit that could function as a CCS and was administered by the Corps Medical Officer – the DDMS.

The MDS also included a Resuscitation Station, and on the Western Front an element of a station for the treatment of gas casualties. The last element of the MDS was the Evacuation Station, from where casualties were evacuated either to a CCS or, when lightly wounded, to a Rest Station.[16]

While the lessons of the Boer War in the area of medical organization at the battlefield were defined and thus could be changed and adjusted to modern warfare, the story of military surgery was quite different. During the first phase of the Boer War military surgeons chose to operate on penetrating abdominal wounds. After quite a short time they were annoyed by their bad results: the post-operative mortality rate was higher than mortality among casualties who had not been operated on at all. As the causes of these results were not understood at the time, surgeons at the various field hospitals ceased to operate on cases of penetrating abdominal wounds. This expectant attitude towards abdominal wounds would remain in effect until 1915.[17]

There were two main reasons for the failure of abdominal surgery during the Boer War. First of all, most battle injuries among British troops were caused by bullets fired from the Mauser rifles in use by the Boer commandos. These 'high velocity' and 'small calibre' bullets caused relatively little damage to the affected tissues. The second reason was that field hospitals were generally located far away from the firing line. Thus, battle casualties suffering from penetrating wounds had to travel long distances over rough terrain in order to undergo an operation. When they reached the operating theatres, many of them were already dying or doomed. The famous surgeon Sir Cuthbert Wallace would write later:

> The reason of want of success is at once obvious: the cases arrived too late. It was not so much the question of the success of the expectant treatment as a failure of the operative [...]. The reason for the late operation was the nature of fighting in an unsettled country of great distances.[18]

These results, especially concerning abdominal wounds, were very annoying:

> [...] it began to be observed that a significant number of patients who had a bullet wound of the abdomen and were left unoperated on recovered without operation. Treves at Colenso described the Mauser bullet as 'a very merciful one.'[19]
>
> So it began to be accepted that no abdominal case required operation, certainly not as a primary laparotomy and only at a later period 'if the symptoms showed that recovery was hopeless in either case, with or without operation.' This assumption continued to be held fourteen years later.[20]

Many years later, Benton would write:

> An unfortunate consequence of the Boer War surgeons' high success rate was the overoptimism carried into World War I. Surgeons in that war soon discovered that much of the Boer War surgical success could be attributed to the types of weapons used as well as to the favourable climatic and environmental conditions of South Africa. The shift from rifles to artillery and the abundance of infectious micro-organisms in European soil forced World War I surgeons again to face the traditional battlefield problem of controlling Sepsis.[21]

The Boer War also marked the establishment of the institution of 'surgical consultants,' so important during the future Great War. It began when several senior civilian surgeons offered their services to the newly formed RAMC which was already engaged in war. When most of the Medical Officers were civilian doctors who generally lacked any knowledge concerning the special aspects of military medicine, the role of the consultants became very important. During the Great War, there were no RAMC rules governing the treatment of various injuries. The task of the consultants was to diffuse recent advances and professional knowledge among the surgeons in the field. In this way, they created a policy concerning the various practical aspects of surgery on the battlefield.[22]

It might be important to note that the surgical lessons of the Russo-Japanese War (1904–05) were quite different from those acquired in the Boer War. The main insight gained from the former demonstrated quite clearly the importance of early operation as the cardinal positive predictive value for operative success. The military-surgical lessons learned from that war were known to the RAMC through senior British Medical Officers who served as observers during that conflict and reported from the battlefield. However they were ignored, and the British preferred to cling to their own lessons gained from the Boer War.[23]

In 1907 a mobile surgical unit was created and given the name 'Clearing Hospital,' one it would retain until January 1915. The Clearing Hospital was intended to receive and provide temporary care for sick and wounded soldiers during their evacuation from the front. Its functions were similar to those of the 'Tent Sub-Division' of the field ambulance.

During the relatively short first phase of the Great War, fighting consisted of speedy movement of military formations. This mode of combat made the process of medical evacuation very difficult, so many cases of penetrating wounds arrived too late at the hospitals, and their prospects of survival, or even of being helped by operative procedures, was very low, as in South Africa. The Clearing Hospital became an essential link between the field ambulance and the rear hospitals.[24]

By the end of 1914 it became obvious that the Clearing Hospital was not the appropriate answer to the surgical problems on the battlefield. Since it did not have any tents or huts and did not include x-rays machines and other essential medical equipment and services, it could not serve as a proper hospital dealing with urgent surgical cases in short time. The causing agent had also changed: most of the casualties were not the result of rifle bullets but rather were caused by fragments of shrapnel and artillery shells. It was also realized that in contrast to the dry and relatively clean South African soil, that of Europe was cultivated and contaminated by tetanus bacilli and other micro-organisms, which contributed to morbidity and mortality among battle casualties. Evaluation of the situation brought about a change in policy towards early operation, which from that time on became the leading attitude toward these cases.

Sir Anthony Bowlby, a surgical consultant at the Western Front, and others devised the concept of a Casualty Clearing Station (CCS). This unit should be a forward surgical centre, located about five miles behind the MDS, manned with professionals and well equipped, in which surgery of urgent cases – especially abdominal cases – would be conducted. The establishment of the CCSs significantly reduced the lag period between wounding and operation, and eventually would save many lives.[25] Of the CCS it has been written:

> The ideal CCS should furnish hospital accommodations for sick and wounded as near the front line as possible, and evacuate those to be taken to the rear as rapidly as possible.
>
> In running the CCS one should always keep in mind that the lines of communication must be kept clear. Ordinarily it should be the object of the CCS to retain all slightly wounded who can return to duty, or, in other words, those who require not more than two weeks treatment, as well as those who can not be moved without risk to life [...].[26]

A CCS was staffed by eight surgeons and anaesthesiologists, and seventy-seven others. It was built to operate on urgent cases of various kinds, in eight teams simultaneously. In addition to the operating theatre, the CCS included a general admission tent, separate tents for the dressing of walking patients and of lying-down patients, a pre-operation tent, a resuscitation tent, and an evacuation tent. It could accommodate 200 casualties at the same time: 50 in beds and 150 on stretchers. On the Western Front, the CCS was located near a railway junction and should have a good road for the transport of incoming and outgoing patients.[27]

The CCS , though allotted per a division, was neither a divisional nor a corps medical unit. This meant that it took orders only from the DMS, unless specified otherwise. It was an immobile unit, not possessing any transport means of its own. When it had to move, it was provided with transportation by the 'Q' branch of the staff. Due to practical considerations the CCS was divided into a 'Light Section' and a 'Heavy Section.' The Light Section could be transported easily when it was necessary to take over an MDS which had to move on with its advancing division. It might also be used at times as an Advanced Operating Centre.

It was the policy of the RAMC that 'every case of wound, no matter how slight, received an injection of 5000 units of anti-tetanic serum. In a base hospital all serious cases would get another such injection.' From 1916 on, most of the operations and blood transfusions were performed at the CCS level.[28] During the '3rd Ypres campaign,' which lasted for three and a half months in 1917, 61,500 operations under anaesthetics were performed in the CCSs of two armies.[29]

From the CCS, casualties were further evacuated to rear hospitals – Stationary Hospitals with 400 beds and General Hospitals having 600, 1040, or 1200 beds. These hospitals were part of the medical units of the 'Lines of Communications' (L-of-C) of an Army. The L-of-C was a system of communication by road, rail, and ships between an Army and its bases. It also included the districts through which they passed.[30] Among the medical units of the L-of- C were Ambulance Trains, a Field Hygiene Section, Convalescent Depots, Hospital Ships, and a Base Depot of Medical Stores.

The RAMC functionaries who were expected to plan and coordinate the treatment and evacuation of casualties from the RAP to the rear hospitals were senior medical officers. The first among them was the Assistant Director of the Medical Services (ADMS), the Medical Officer at the division level. His rank was usually that of Colonel or Lt-Colonel in the RAMC He commanded all the RAMC personnel in a division: those of the three field ambulances, the sanitary sections, and also the RAMC officers and other ranks in all the divisional units except the battalions. He was assisted by a Deputy Assistant Director of the Medical Services (DADMS). The ADMS was responsible for all arrangements concerning the collection and evacuation of the sick and wounded from the RAPs to the corresponding subdivisions of the field ambulance, the ADS and the DMS.[31] This included the selection of suitable sites for those stations and the reconnoitering of all routes which might serve for evacuation of casualties to the various medical echelons. The ADMS was also charged with issuing the 'Medical Operation Order' after receiving the Division Operational Orders and with preparation of a Medical Paragraph for insertion in the Divisional Administrative Order. It was his responsibility to secure a reserve of stretchers and blankets for divisional needs and received reports from all OC Field Ambulances every 4–6 hours. He was also the commander of the Divisional Sanitary Section and responsible for its professional activities.[32]

The Medical Officer of an Army Corps was the Deputy Director of the Medical Services (DDMS). He held the rank of Colonel in the RAMC and was responsible for the evacuation of casualties from the divisions, mainly from MDSs to CCSs. This was generally executed by the Motor Ambulance Convoy, which was operated by the DDMS. Under his direct command were only the Corps Field Ambulance and the Corps Hygiene Section. The Corps Field Ambulance was a Corps reserve medical unit which was used by the DDMS in order to assist divisional field ambulances at times of pressure. It could be used also as a Corps MDS when necessary. When several divisions were attacking on a narrow front, a Corps MDS might be preferable to divisional arrangements according to the Corps medical plan. The DDMS was also responsible for holding conferences of the Corps ADMSs and the commanders of field ambulances.[33]

A Motor Ambulance Convoy was allotted to every Corps. It consisted of seventy-five motor ambulances organized in three sections; a fourth section being a workshop. Its importance was especially at times when railway communications broke down or were insufficient.

The Director of Army Medical Services, the Medical Officer at an Army HQ, was the DMS. He was a very senior RAMC figure, usually holding the rank of Major General and with the status of a Surgeon General in the hierarchy of the RAMC. His main task was to supervise the work of the medical services in the Army area. He was responsible for the arrangements for the evacuation of casualties from the CCSs to rear hospitals – Base and General, usually by Hospital Trains.[34] At times of active fighting his main concern was the work at the CCSs and the distribution of casualties in the L-of-C and base areas.[35]

Both the DDMS and the DMS were responsible for the sanitary organization in their respective formations. The process of evacuation between the field ambulance and the CCS was controlled either by the Corps DDMS or an Army DMS, according to the scenario.[36]

During 1916, when the Egyptian Expeditionary Force (EEF) was gradually leaving the Canal Zone and penetrating into the Sinai Desert, it included an experienced medical service. This service was organized according to the lessons acquired on the Western Front, which had transformed the RAMC of

1914 into a well- established, professional, and efficient service. It included many Medical Officers, of all ranks, who had acquired much experience on various battlefields, mainly in France and the Dardanelles. It also included field ambulances and surgical units which had served on the Western Front, at Macedonia, and at Gallipoli.

There were several differences between the European and Egyptian fronts. Medical officers at the higher levels realized that they could expect a battleground in which the main health issues might be mobile warfare with no real routes for evacuation of casualties, lack of water, and infectious diseases. The surgical teams which had gained their experience either in France or in Gallipoli were surprised at the remarkable absence of gas gangrene due to the nature of the soil, as in South Africa.[37] The cavalry divisions' medical services faced some changes in their organization: the traditional field ambulance consisting of three sections was transformed into a more compact unit. It consisted of one HQ Section, one Mobile Section, and two Mobile Convoys. The HQ Section formed an MDS and also carried equipment for establishing an ADS. According to Colonel R.M. Downes, the DDMS of the EEF Desert Mounted Corps, the modus operandi too had undergone considerable change:

> Though the textbook teaching visualized the Field Ambulance as carrying out most of the collection of wounded after the action was over, this was not the method usually adopted. Instead, wounded were collected as soon as possible, and while as many as could be were sent back on their horses or walked, the main object was to bring up the ambulance transport as far forward as possible to the collecting posts or even the firing line whenever there was sufficient cover.[38]

The Sinai Desert and Palestine would be a totally new military experience. Naturally it demanded and deserved different military medicine than that practiced at that time on the Western Front.

2

THE DESERT CAMPAIGNS: FROM THE SUEZ CANAL TO THE GATES OF GAZA, 1915–1917

'The advance across the Sinai desert, therefore, may well be described as a triumph of the engineering and medical services over disease.'

William G. Macpherson, *History of the Great War, Based on Official Documents: Medical Services – General History*, vol. 3 (London: HMSO, 1924), 435.

'The work of the MC and the Stretcher Bearers was again magnificent. The little canvas hooded sand-carts were to be seen on all part of the field throughout the action, approaching right up to the firing-line again and again.'

Charles G. Powles, *The New Zealanders in Sinai and Palestine* (Auckland: Withcombe and Tombs, 1922), 78.

On 5 November 1914 the Ottoman Empire – Turkey – joined Germany and the Central Alliance in the war against the Entente Powers. This act endangered both the Suez Canal as a vital marine route and control of the oil fields in the Persian Gulf area. On 6 November a British division, sent from India, landed at Shat el-Arab. This force took the important town of Basra on 22 November and secured the area of the oil fields by capturing Kurna on 9 December 1914.

In Egypt the situation was quite different. There, British forces had been present and involved in various aspects of Egyptian politics for a long time, since 'the safety of the Suez Canal was of such importance to the British Empire at war that military and political control of Egypt had to be retained in some shape or other.'[1]

The shapers of Ottoman Empire strategy were very much aware of the importance of the Suez Canal for the British Empire. They realized that creating a permanent threat against the canal zone would compel the British to defend Egypt with large forces. In the grand strategy of the Central Alliance this meant that British forces would be diverted from other fronts in order to protect Egypt, a diversion which might contribute to various German–Turkish military plans. Already in 1914 Turkish military units occupied two key points in the Sinai Peninsula: El Arish and Nekhl. Both were remote from the Canal itself and their garrisons served mainly as a declaration of threat against it.

British strategy in the Middle East, at least during the initial phase of the war, was purely defensive, with the objective of securing intact functioning of the Suez Canal at all times: 'The task of the defence, however, was not merely to bar the road to Egypt, but to ensure every portion of the Canal from damage or destruction.'[2] Thus, during the first months of the war the British garrison in Egypt was rather small, to be replaced later by a Territorial Division. When the British intelligence noticed Turkish formations being concentrated in Palestine and Syria, it was decided to train the Australian and New Zealand regiments in Egypt, on their way to the Western Front. In this manner the garrison was augmented by these mounted units. Since September 1914 the British forces in Egypt were commanded by General John Maxwell, a capable administrator who knew Egypt very well and was well versed in the specific political problems of the area. As a military commander he saw his task as being strictly defensive and static: British units defended the Suez Canal upon its banks.[3]

The British defensive plan was also based on firm geographical considerations: between the Suez Canal and the Turkish army, which was concentrated in Palestine and in Syria, lay many miles of desert of the Sinai Peninsula. The Sinai desert seemed to be a prominent natural obstacle for any aggressor attempting to approach the Suez Canal from the east. Very few routes could serve a Turkish military advance through Sinai, and lack of water would limit the size and tactical options of any unit trying to cross the desert in the direction of the canal.

In January 1915 a Turkish expeditionary force under the command of

Djemal Pasha and his chief of staff, the German Colonel Friedrich Kress von Kressenstein, crossed the Sinai desert, unnoticed during most of its advance, and reached the Suez Canal with the intention of capturing the canal area and arousing a civil uprising against the British in Egypt. The raid was the result of careful planning and meticulous preparation: water tanks had been buried and scattered along various routes the future raiding force would take and several of the routes had been improved for transport of artillery and heavy logistic equipment. All these preparations in the desert, a prerequisite for the raid's success, had passed unnoticed by British intelligence. The Turkish raiding force included about 22,000 troops supported by artillery and logistic units.

Kress von Kressenstein, the mastermind behind the daring raid, was a unique commander who cared for his soldiers at all times. He knew that a raiding force should be self-sustained and considered the care of sick and wounded to be a crucial issue. Thus, the raiding force included three field ambulances and two medical companies capable of caring for hundreds of casualties during a day, pending on being re-supplied with dressings and medical equipment. Casualties would be initially treated and stabilized hemodynamically at a medical company, and then be evacuated to one of the mobile field hospitals where they would receive advanced treatment. For casualties in need of an urgent operation, this could be performed at the level of the field hospital.[4]

The Turkish raiding force left southern Palestine on 15 January 1915, reaching the Suez Canal on 3 February, which it began to cross. When the Turkish attackers approached the canal they were at last spotted by the British defenders. The battle was very short – the raiders were repulsed and pushed back into the Sinai desert, suffering heavy losses. No British unit pursued the Turkish raiding force, which beat a fairly organized retreat to Palestine. Though the Turkish raid against the Suez Canal failed completely, it demonstrated to the British high command in Egypt that defence of the Canal Zone, and of Egypt in general, could not be based solely on natural obstacles such as the Sinai desert and the Canal.

By early 1915 British strategy in Egypt had changed and was no longer limited to defence of the canal. By the end of 1914 the situation at the war's main front, the European Western Front, became static. The opposing troops formed constant lines of trenches and barbed wire in which they were entrenched. This was a veritable deadlock.

Several British statesmen and generals began to believe that the Turkish participation in the war might serve as a lever to solve the problem of the European deadlock. They thought that knocking Turkey out of the war would bring the Balkan States to support the Entente and also create such an imbalance that would eventually lead to victory over Germany in Europe. It was therefore advocated that Britain's main military initiative should be shifted from Europe to the Middle East, where British forces could attack the Ottoman Empire at strategic and vulnerable places. The main protagonists of this attitude were, among others, the statesman David Lloyd George, Field Marshal Lord Kitchener, and First Lord of the Admiralty Winston Churchill. Should such a plan materialize, it would be under the command of the HQ British Expeditionary Force in Egypt, which would then become the Mediterranean Expeditionary Force.

It should be borne in mind that throughout the war there was a debate among policy makers and strategists in London. The Chief of the Imperial General Staff at that time, Sir William Robertson, and others were of the opinion that the outcome of the war against Germany would be determined only on the Western Front, for which they earned the sobriquet 'Westerners.' They considered any other battlefield a 'side show.' Others thought that due to the stalemate on the Western Front only a thrust against Germany's chief alley, i.e., Turkey, in the Middle East, might produce favourable results. These statesmen, naturally, were called 'Easterners.'

The objective selected was the Gallipoli Peninsula, not far from Constantinople, the capital of the Ottoman Empire, and controlling the Dardanelles, an obligatory marine passage between the Black Sea and the Mediterranean. On 25 April 1915 British forces landed at the Gallipoli Peninsula. From the very first they faced strong Turkish resistance and for long months were checked not far from the shores on which they had landed. During the long months between April 1915 and 8 January 1916, when they eventually evacuated Gallipoli without any real military gain, the British forces sustained about 200,000 casualties: 115,000 battle casualties and 85,000 sick soldiers who had to be evacuated.[5]

While medical treatment at the regimental level and at the field ambulances was the best which could be tendered under the circumstances, medical evacuation on board boats as well as the command and coordination of the medical evacuation process were deficient. This was the result of several factors.

According to the attitude of Sir Ian Hamilton, commander of the British forces in the Dardanelles campaign, and his staff officers, there was no need to involve the DMS in its planning. During the campaign itself the medical services operated mostly on their own, without any involvement or help from the relevant staff officers. Another problem lay in the medical services themselves: Surgeon General R.W. Ford was the senior medical officer in Egypt, his title being DMS, Egypt. Thus, theoretically he was the senior medical officer during the campaign. However, Surgeon General W.G. Bedford was the DMS of the Expeditionary Force to the Dardanelles, Surgeon General W.G. Birrell was DMS at the island of Imbros, where most of the medical facilities were located during the campaign and to which the majority of the sick and wounded were evacuated, and Colonel John Maher was the DDMS of the L-of-C. The hierarchy and linkage among all these functionaries had never been defined, nor their exact tasks and responsibilities. Naturally this situation served as a source of friction and misunderstanding.

The troops who fought in the Gallipoli Peninsula suffered from several diseases. What was common to all these diseases was the fact that they could all be prevented by simple measures – proper behaviour of the troops and support of the commanders in the field. Flies that fed on corpses left in the open transmitted contagious diseases of the gastrointestinal tract. Various micro-organisms were transmitted directly from one soldier to another due to lack of basic personal and camp hygiene. Thus, soldiers suffered from dysentery, both bacillary and amoebic, infective jaundice, typhoid, and paratyphoid fever. During August and September 1915 as many as 78 percent of the troops were suffering from dysentery or other intestinal diseases. At the same time 64 percent suffered from septic sores, a secondary skin infection typical of people who were deprived of basic hygienic measures, suffered from malnutrition, or both. At an advanced stage of the campaign soldiers began indeed to suffer from deficiency diseases such as beri-beri and scurvy due to failure to supply the frontline soldiers with adequate food. It is of interest that there were no cases of cholera due to the fact that all soldiers had been inoculated against that disease as a prophylactic measure.

Late 1915 and early 1916 were a nadir in the condition of the British Empire in the Middle East. While British forces were involved in aimless battle in Gallipoli, another British failure was on its way in the Middle East. In Mesopotamia, a British offensive was mounted along the Tigris River, in the direction of the important city of Baghdad, by the 6th Division under the command of General Charles Townshend. The beginning was very promising

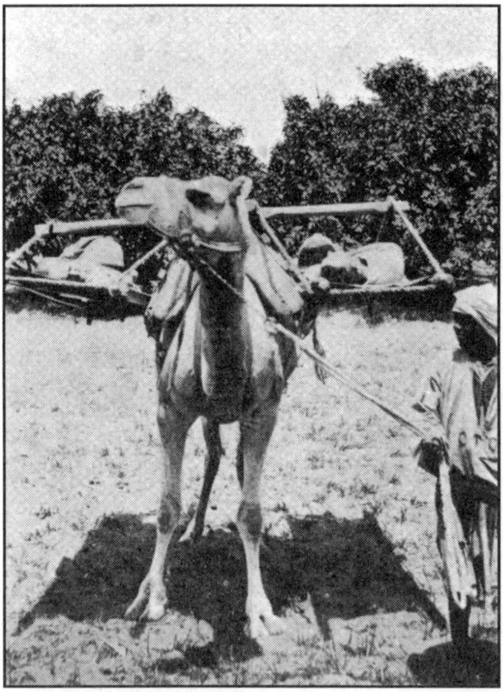

An improved cacolet for patients lying down

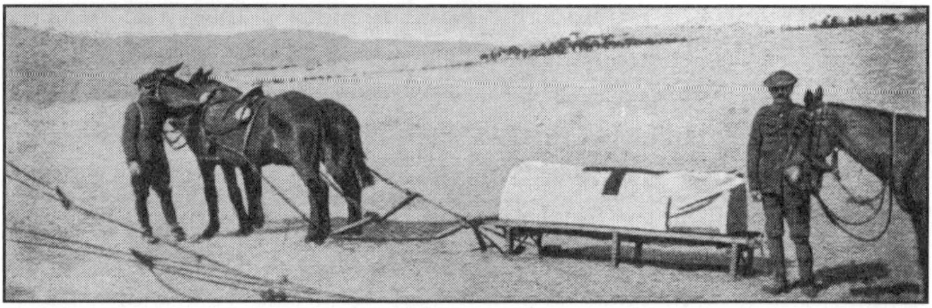

An ambulance sledge

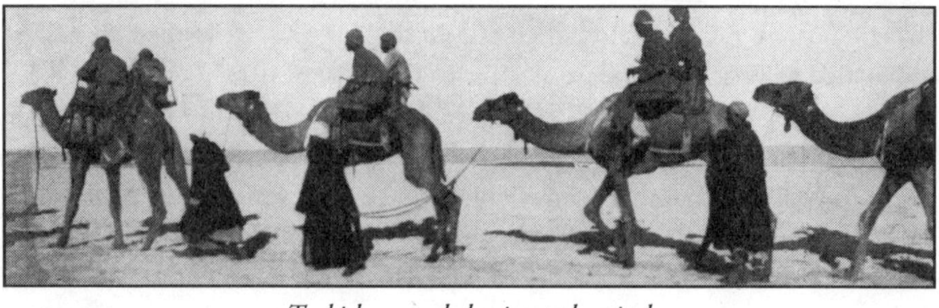

Turkish wounded going to hospital

as the division dashed towards Baghdad with almost no opposition. However, it outstretched its lines of communications to a point that maintenance of the force became almost impossible. This thrust was checked by the Turks at Ctesiphon, not far from Baghdad.

At the battle of Ctesiphon, on 22 November 1915, the 6th Division suffered 4,593 casualties, about 30 percent of the force. Unable to proceed in the direction of Baghdad, the division retreated to Kut-el-Amara, where it came under siege by superior Turkish forces. Evacuation of the casualties from the battle of Ctesiphon was a total failure due to bad planning. Several British attempts to raise the siege and release the 6th Division failed, their cost in human lives being very high: over 40,000 casualties.

The 6th Division was besieged at Kut-el-Amara from 5 December 1915 until 29 April 1916. During that lengthy period the besieged troops suffered from a variety of diseases, mainly dysentery and malaria, but also from typhoid and paratyphoid fever. Due to the breakdown of the logistic systems, there was a severe shortage of food and drinking water. Soldiers began to suffer from deficiency diseases, mainly the Indian troops who were vegetarians and did not consume flesh of horses when it came to that point. Cases of beri-beri and scurvy, due to vitamin deficiency, were quite common. By the end of April 1916 there were almost no food reserves left. On 29 April 1916 General Townshend and his garrison of 2,750 British and 6,500 Indian troops, surrendered to the superior Turkish force which had besieged them and marched into captivity.[6]

The double British defeat in the Dardanelles and in Mesopotamia did not go unnoticed in public opinion: national enquiry commissions were appointed in both cases and their conclusions and recommendations were publicized. The Mesopotamia Commission Report, published in August 1917, dealt with the operations in Mesopotamia prior to July 1916 and described what had happened as a 'medical breakdown.' In both cases it became obvious that among other deficiencies in planning, command, and control, the medical aspects of those campaigns had been ignored and health issues had not been a part of the planning and of the appraisement of the situation.

The defeat of the two British expeditionary forces, in the Dardanelles and in Mesopotamia, was not only a blow at British prestige in the Near East; it also put an end for a time to any real hope of rapidly getting Turkey out of the war.

On 10 January 1916 Sir John Maxwell, the commanding officer of the

British troops in Egypt, was succeeded by Sir Archibald Murray as commander of the British forces at the Suez Canal Front. In March General Murray became sole commander of the British troops in Egypt which from 19 March would be known as The Egyptian Expeditionary Force (EEF). Surgeon General Ford left Egypt at that time to be succeeded as DMS EEF by Colonel John Maher.

On 15 February 1916 General Murray sent to the Chief of the Imperial General Staff (CIGS) his thoughts concerning the defence of the Canal Zone:

> [...] the passive defence of the Canal was very wasteful of men and material [...]. Strategically, therefore, the true base of the defensive zone of Egypt against invasion from the east is not the 80 or 90 miles of the Canal Zone, but the 45 miles between El Arish and El Kossaima. [...] From the point of view of the permanent security of Egypt, therefore, it is highly desirable that El Arish should be occupied by us with mobile forces of sufficient size. [...] If El Arish could be held, the permanent occupation of other points in the Sinai Peninsula outside the Canal Zone, would appear to be unnecessary.[7]

As a result of this new attitude, mounted troops were bivouacking in the desert, east of the Suez Canal. They began to reconnoitre the western part of the Sinai desert, with mounted units reaching central Sinai quite frequently. After the Dardanelles campaign, most of the troops from Australia and New Zealand were sent to France, where they formed two ANZAC Corps. The brigades that were left in Egypt – the 1st, 2nd, and 3rd Australian Light Horse Brigades and the New Zealand Mounted Rifles Brigade – formed the ANZAC Mounted Division under General Harry Chauvel. Lt-Col. Rupert M. Downes, who had served in the Dardanelles campaign as commander of the 3rd Light Horse Field Ambulance, was appointed ADMS of the new division. The DADMS of the new division was Capt. Charles E. Hercus.

General Murray began to build a standard gauge railway and parallel to it a 12-inch water pipeline which would bring drinking water from the sweet water canal in Egypt to the Sinai desert. These two monumental projects would enable British troops to cross the desert. General Murray's future successor, Field Marshal Edmund Allenby, when summing up the Palestine campaigns in 1919, would in his last despatch recall Murray's two projects, which had been a prerequisite to the successful Palestine campaigns:

> I desire to express my indebtedness to my predecessor, Lieutenant-General Sir A.J. Murray, who, by his bridging of the desert between Egypt and Palestine, laid the foundations for the subsequent advances of the Egyptian Expeditionary Force. I reaped the fruits of his foresight and strategical imagination, which brought the waters of the Nile to the borders of Palestine, planned the skilful military operations by which the Turks were driven from strong positions in the desert over the frontier of Egypt, and carried a standard gauge railway to the gates of Gaza. The organization he created, both in Sinai and in Egypt, stood all tests and formed the corner-stone of my successes.[8]

In the meantime, during the spring and summer of 1916 the ANZAC and the yeomanry units were responsible for the security of the railway, the pipeline, and their workers. The Turkish intelligence was aware of the British change in attitude concerning the defence of the Canal.

One of the places in Sinai around which mounted units were located was Qatiya, an oasis in the western Sinai desert whose wells could supply high quality drinking water either to British units defending the Canal or to Turkish units on their way to the Canal.

On 23 April 1916, a well-planned Turkish assault took a yeomanry unit at Qatiya by surprise. The attack lasted for two days and ended when the British troops in the area, who suffered severe casualties, abandoned their positions and retreated in the direction of the Suez Canal.[9] The lessons of the Turkish attack on Qatiya were well studied on several levels. First of all, the incident contributed much to the understanding of every unit in Sinai that it might be the object of a surprise attack at any moment. The locations and movements of the various mounted units now became more coordinated so that units under attack could expect to be reinforced and helped in due time by others in the area. It was also understood that every mounted unit in the desert should be augmented by medical personnel, as their ability to provide proper treatment at the front before evacuation to medical installations might be crucial to the condition of the casualties.

During the first years of the war the medical services of the British

Expeditionary Force in Egypt included only the field ambulances which had arrived at Egypt with the units themselves. Sick and wounded soldiers who were treated at these medical installations were further evacuated to Egyptian civilian hospitals. This situation remained unchanged until January 1916, after the Dardanelles Campaign. At that time, several hospitals arrived in Egypt to join the forces there. Thus, in February 1916 there was a real medical, surgical, and hospitalization system in eastern Egypt and the canal zone. At Port Said, where the Suez Canal opens into the Mediterranean Sea, were located No. 31 General Hospital, No. 15 Stationary Hospital, No. 26 CCS, a sanitary section, an advanced depot of medical stores, and a bacteriological laboratory. There were a CCS (No. 54) and a sanitary section at Qantara. At Feirdan, further to the south and nearer the Canal, were another CCS (No. 24) and an additional sanitary section. The No. 2 Australian Stationary Hospital was at El Kebir, while at the Ismailia area were located No. 1 Australian Stationary Hospital, the New Zealand Stationary Hospital, Nos. 1 and 2 Australian CCSs, and two sections of the No. 124 Indian Combined Field Ambulance.[10]

In April 1916, Colonel John Maher, who served as the DDMS L-of-C during the Gallipoli Campaign, succeeded Surgeon General W.G. Bedford, who had been invalided back to England. This coincided with the departure of Surgeon General Ford from Egypt. At last there was only one DMS in the area who was responsible for all medical and health services in Egypt. His HQ was located at Ismailia, in the canal zone. His ADMS was Colonel A.E.C. Keble and his ADMS for sanitation was Colonel C.H. Melville. When Surgeon General Maher entered upon his new post he found a well organized military medical system which included 11,162 hospital beds and 4,646 beds for convalescents.

The cardinal difficulty facing the medical system concerned the evacuation of casualties from the firing line to the dressing stations due to the lack of portable stretchers designed for cavalry casualties. Several creative solutions were found. The first was *cacolets*, specially designed seats on both sides of a camel, known already to Napoleon's surgeon Dominique Jean Larrey who had served in Napoleon's Palestine campaigns in 1799–1800. They were useful for both sitting and lying casualties. The other solutions for medical evacuation in the desert were sand carts and sand sledges.[11]

The sand or desert carts, officially known as 'desert ambulance carts,' were carts on wheels drawn either by camels or by mules and especially designed for conveyance of two casualties with minimum inconvenience caused by the motion of the cart. They were used mainly for transport from Advanced Dressing Stations and Main Dressing Stations of cases of abdominal wounds, femoral fractures, etc.[12] Sand sledges were platforms especially designed for carrying sick and wounded soldiers over dunes and sandy terrain. Their great advantage was their ability to carry casualties over sand, where no cart or vehicle on wheels could move without sinking in the sand.[13] The 'Maltese Cart' was 'a square contrivance on two wheels and no springs, drawn by three horses abreast.'[14]

The field ambulances in the Sinai desert differed from the usual field ambulances: they included only two sections instead of three, with the addition of thirty-six stretcher-bearers and three officers. The 'C' sections, which were separated from their eight original units, were organized in order to form new medical units. Another innovation was the addition of a dental section to each field ambulance.[15] By the end of January 1916 the field ambulances had been supplied with *cacolet*s and sand carts.[16]

The Turks tried their luck again at Romani on 4 August 1916, the battle lasting for ten days until 14 August. However, this time the outcome was completely different than that which had been experienced previously at Qatiya: the mounted troops could take their revenge on the aggressors, as they had been expected. According to the 'Official History' of the Great War: 'Romani was a considerable British victory. The enemy completely failed in his object and lost nearly four thousand prisoners. [...] The British casualties were 1130 with a low proportion of killed and a very small proportion of missing.'[17] The enemy suffered about 9,000 casualties out of a force of 18,000. About 4,000 Turkish troops were taken prisoner and two field ambulances were captured.

Archibald P. Wavell, the future historian of the Palestine campaigns, noted a change in the military situation: 'The victory at Romani marked a turning point in the campaigns based on Egypt. Henceforward that country and the Canal were safe from Turkish attack. From now till the end of the war the British were the aggressors in this theatre.'[18] However, at that time the change was only a tactical and not a strategic one, as the War Cabinet had not yet made up its mind considering the strategy and future conduct of the war in the Middle East. That period of time was typical of the undefined and ever-changing British strategy.[19]

The medical units of the ANZAC Mounted Division and the Yeomanry

Brigade were well organized for the battle at Romani by the ADMS ANZAC Division Lt-Col. Rupert Downes. The mobile sections of the field ambulances of the Light Horse Brigades followed their units, each augmented by eight sand carts carried by mules for evacuation of battle casualties. The mobile sections formed ADSs for their brigades close to the firing line. Casualties were evacuated from these ADSs to the tent sub-division of the field ambulances which stayed behind to form MDSs. No.3 Field Ambulance of the 42nd (Lowland) Division, which was also in the area, formed a CCS at the railhead at Romani, to where all casualties were eventually evacuated. A Turkish field hospital captured during the battle of Romani was immediately put into operation, its task being the treatment of Turkish casualties. Battle casualties of the 42nd and the 52nd Divisions, which also participated in the battle, were evacuated to the rear by camel convoys. As one authoritative source reports: 'During the battle of Romani no hospital trains were sent east of the Canal and the casualties had to be evacuated on open trucks by the light railway from Mahamdiyah to Port Said and from Romani to Qantara.'[20]

During September 1916 an Eastern Force of the EEF was formed under the command of Lt-Gen. Sir Charles Dobell. It took command of all British units east of the Suez Canal, with HQ at Ismailia. As a result, the DMS and his HQ moved from Ismailia back to Cairo, where the GHQ of the EEF was located. Colonel M.J. Sexton was assigned as DDMS Eastern Force and moved to Ismailia. His DADMS was Captain J.H. Wood. Colonel C.J. Macdonald, formerly the DDMS of one of the sections of the Canal, who had 'considerable experience of warfare in France,' became DDMS Desert Column, the mobile force of the Eastern Force, under the command of Lt.-General Sir Philip Chetwode. His ADMS for sanitation was Major Percy S. Lelean.[21] Colonel Macdonald was highly respected by General Chetwode who 'kept him fully informed of his plans in advance.'[22]

All this changed in December 1916 when David Lloyd George, who since 7 July 1916 had been the Secretary of State for War, succeeded Mr Asquith as Britain's Prime Minister. Lloyd George was a true 'Easterner' who believed that knocking Turkey out of the war would significantly influence the situation at the Western Front. As a result, one of his first actions was to cable General Murray that 'successes in the East were much required.'[23]

At that time the British railway reached El Mazar, not far from El Arish. It enabled Chetwode's Desert Column of the Eastern Force to advance towards that town, the capital of Sinai and the key for the defence of the Canal Zone from the East. The medical services of the Eastern Force, and of the EEF in general, were well prepared for the expected battle of El Arish. Six squads of stretcher bearers were allotted to every brigade. As at the battle of Romani, the mobile sections of the various field ambulances would serve as ADSs while the immobile sections would be amalgamated in order to serve as a CCS, with 700 beds, at the most remote railhead. No. 24 CCS (400 beds) moved from Feirdan at the Canal to Bir el Abed; No. 26 CCS (400 beds) moved from Port Said to El Mazar; No. 54 CCS (200 beds) moved from Qantara to the railhead to be joined by No. 53 CCS from Egypt (200 beds). No. 24 Stationary Hospital (800 beds) moved from Moasacar to Qantara-East while No. 2 Stationary Hospital (800 beds) came from Port Said to be located at Mahamdiyah. Thus, altogether, on the eve of the expected battle of El Arish there were 3,500 beds and all the corresponding medical and surgical facilities, ready to receive casualties. Two hospital trains, Nos. 6 and 7, were also ready to transport casualties.[24]

On 21 December 1916 the Desert Column reached El Arish and the troops were amazed to find that the Turkish garrison, believed to consist of 1,600 well trained and entrenched troops, had evacuated it. Immediately the place became a front base for future operations. The next operation took place almost immediately: from reports by Royal Flying Corps (RFC) pilots it became apparent that the majority of the troops who had fled from El Arish were on their way to Magdhaba, about twenty-five miles southeast of El Arish on the banks of Wadi El Arish. The British realized that Magdhaba had been prepared as a fortified post and included a system of five well constructed redoubts. General Chetwode decided not to allow the enemy to reorganize at Magdhaba and to attack the retreating Turkish force as soon as possible. It was also remembered that Magdhaba, together with Rafah, were the last Turkish garrisons in the Sinai Peninsula. The political significance of capturing these two was that British forces would be at the southern gates of Palestine.

The British force assigned to this mission was commanded by General Chauvel and consisted of the ANZAC Mounted Division (the 1st and 3rd Australian Light Horse Brigades and the New Zealand Mounted Rifles Brigade), the Imperial Camel Corps Brigade, and artillery batteries. General Chetwode was aware that the force was expected to attack a Turkish stronghold quite far inland from the coast, where most of the logistic and medical facilities were located. Thus, he kept the DDMS Desert Column, Colonel

C.J. Macdonald, informed of all the details of his plan. While the DDMS was responsible for the overall medical plan for the operation, planning the treatment and the evacuation of casualties during the fighting at Magdhaba itself was entrusted to Colonel Rupert Downes, ADMS ANZAC Mounted Division.

All three brigades of the ANZAC Mounted Division had their own field ambulances. However, the Imperial Camel Corps Brigade had no medical unit attached to it. In order to solve this problem, the DDMS Desert Column allocated the 1/1st Welsh Field Ambulance of the 53rd Division for that brigade. Its personnel were mounted on camels, carrying forty-eight spare *cacolets* and nine sand carts. In addition, every Camel Corps company was reinforced by a pair of *cacolets* and a medical orderly.[25] The force was joined on its march by the mobile sections of all participating brigades' field ambulances.[26]

General Chauvel's force reached Magdhaba at dawn on 23 December, after a whole night's ride along Wadi El Arish. The troops approached Magdhaba unnoticed and assaulted the stronghold from all directions. Though the Turkish garrison was surprised, its soldiers fought well and the battle lasted from dawn to the late afternoon. Only then did the defenders give up and surrendered to the ANZACS. The British losses were 146, including 22 dead. 1,282 Turkish officers and soldiers were taken prisoner. A dressing station was established three miles west of Magdhaba by the mobile section of the New Zealand Field Ambulance and the 1st Australian Light Horse Brigade Field Ambulance. Two Australian official histories report the following:

> There had been few casualties at the dressing station up to 2 p.m., but by four o'clock large numbers of wounded were coming in as a result of the final assault. Many of the wounded, both Turkish and British, were brought into the well equipped Turkish Field Hospital at Magdhaba, and as they could not be cleared that night, remained there until the 24th in charge of 3rd Light Horse Field Ambulance.[27]
>
> Shortly after noon of the 24 December, all were sent to the dressing station, whence at 5 p.m. the ambulance convoy set out on its twenty-three miles' march to the receiving station. The night was pitch dark and wet, and the great majority of

> cases were perforce carried in the camel cacolets, which gave great trouble. After nine hours of intense discomfort the convoys were met, a few miles from El Arish, by sand carts- lent once more by the 52nd Division – in which the wounded traveled in comfort to the receiving station, where they arrived at 4 a.m. of December 25th. [...] Here some major surgery was carried out, though with very inadequate appliances. On December 26th a convoy of sandcarts was collected by the ADMS with the intention of evacuating to railhead, but preparations had in the meantime been made by the DDMS for evacuation by sea. Weather, however, did not permit of this, and, after a wait of two days for the sea to subside, orders were received to evacuate to railhead, where a hospital train would receive the wounded. On December 29th the largest single ambulance convoy organized in the campaign, made up of seventy-seven sandcarts, nine sledges, and a number of cacolet camels, moved out in three lines along the beach with 150 wounded. All but a few, too bad to move, were evacuated on the following day to Qantara.[28]

The action at Magdhaba would be remembered as an excellent example of how to exploit mounted troops against isolated fortified posts in an open arena.

When the Turkish fortified post at Rafah was captured by ANZAC mounted units on 9 January 1917, the entire Sinai Peninsula was in British hands. The tactics employed during the capture of Rafah were quite similar to that used previously at Magdhaba. British losses at Rafah totalled 487, including 71 dead. The medical services of the ANZAC Mounted Division were well organized before the action in Rafah. Each field ambulance consisted of 10 pairs of litters, 15 pairs of *cacolets*, 12 sand carts, 12 cycle stretchers, and 6 sand sledges. Such a field ambulance could evacuate 92 casualties at one time.[29] 'The work of the MC and the Stretcher Bearers was again magnificent. The little canvas hooded sand-carts were to be seen on all parts of the field throughout the action, approaching right up to the firing-line again and again.'[30]

On 4 January 1917 the railway reached El Arish to be followed four days later by the pipeline. In addition, a new division was formed out of three

Yeomanry brigades of the EEF, which had not been mounted since their return from the Dardanelles. This new division would participate in the future Palestine campaign as the 74th (Yeomanry) Division. British troops were now stationed at the southern border of Palestine awaiting further orders.

Though the whole Sinai Peninsula was now in British hands, there were still a few Turkish outposts in the heart of the Sinai desert which British patrols had not yet encountered. One of them was Bir el Hassana, situated on Wadi El Arish, about thirty-three miles south of Magdhaba. On 17 February 1917, the 2nd Battalion of the Imperial Camel Corps Brigade, under the command of Major J.R. Bassett, advanced from Magdhaba during the night and surprised the Turkish garrison at Bir el Hassana, which surrendered without any resistance. However, local Bedouins, probably disturbed by the British force, opened fire in its direction. One soldier, Lance-Corporal MacGregor, was injured in his ankle. As the battalion at Bir el Hassana was far away from any other British unit and it had only one casualty, who could not ride on a camel due to the nature of his injury, he was evacuated by a British B.E.2c aeroplane from Bir el Hassana directly to the hospital at El Arish. This case of aero-medical evacuation was unique: except for very rare cases of rescue and air-evacuation of pilots by their comrades, there was no other such case throughout the Palestine campaigns.[31]

During the long stay and the various operations in the Sinai desert, the health of the troops was on the whole very good.[32] Venereal diseases, which had posed a major problem while the troops had been staying in Egypt, practically disappeared in Sinai.[33] The most prevalent disease among the troops was bacillary dysentery, and even it did not appear in an epidemic form. There were sporadic cases of malaria, both in Egypt and later on at the area of Wadi Ghazze near Gaza. All malaria cases at that time were caused by plasmodium vivax. Malaria did not present a real health problem to the troops before entering Palestine itself. Sporadic cases of typhoid fever were noticed occasionally, though most of the troops had been inoculated against this disease. There were also occasional cases of sand-fly fever. These diseases never became a real threat to the health of the troops.

Though all troops had been vaccinated against cholera, it was one of few conditions feared by all. In fact there were several outbreaks of diarrhea suspected as being due to cholera. Though in most of them this was ruled out, yet fear of this disease was deep and might be blamed for unverified rumours, such as the following:

> At El Abd a notice was printed up above two sick Turks: 'Attention! Cholera, with the compliments of the German Ambulance Corps.' A phial [vial] was picked up at Geeila Oasis, containing live cholera germs from a Berlin laboratory. We don't know if they were intended to pollute the water or not. Naturally we are uneasy.[34]

The only medical problem which affected many soldiers, and at times even jeopardized their performance, was that of 'septic' or 'desert' sores:

> It was found that the slightest scratch quickly developed into an intractable ulcer which, in spite of all treatment, would last for months, and nothing seemed to do any good except to send the patient down the line to Egypt, when, with fresh food and vegetables and ordinary simple dressing, the sores quickly healed. The usual explanation offered was that the condition was a food deficiency disease aggravated by sand and heat, and the dietary was accordingly augmented by vegetables as fresh as possible [...].[35]

Apparently there was a debate between the doctors concerning the cause of this disease and how to cope with it: 'DDMS supports a request from the Desert Column to purchase oranges due to septic sores; it is denied. 1 ton costs 15 shillings and they will need 15 ton/day. DMS thinks it is not obligatory as infection is not nutritional but due to circumstances.'[36]

While the troops were entrenched around Gaza, an epidemic of desert sores in their ranks was accompanied by an outbreak of a mild form of diphtheria. Captain C.M. Craig of No. 2 Military Laboratory, stationed at Deir el Belah, who tried to study the nature of the bacteriological origin of the sores, found that many of them gave a positive culture of diphtheroids. This observation was later confirmed by other laboratory methods. It led to the practice of injecting anti-diphtheric serum to soldiers who suffered from sores and this was 'found to be of therapeutic value.'[37]

While at the gates of Palestine, General Murray took two decisions, the first being to advance into Palestine along the coastline. The second was to act swiftly, as he was afraid that the enemy 'should evacuate Gaza and withdraw out of reach before a blow could be struck on him.'[38]

The First Battle of Gaza began on 26 March 1917. Morning fog delayed the attack and the 'enveloping' of the town was achieved only by evening. At that time, General Charles Dobbel, the commander of the Eastern Force, who was the officer commanding the forces attacking Gaza, was worried about an incipient counterattack by superior enemy forces expected to arrive from the northeast. Due to lack of real-time intelligence, Dobell was not aware of the desperate situation of the defenders and decided that 'unless Gaza was captured by nightfall the fight must be broken off and the mounted troops withdrawn.' Several misunderstandings created an uncoordinated withdrawal from the town which had practically been captured.

After the First Battle of Gaza, one of the officers participating in it made the following notation in his diary:

> [...] we got into the Turkish positions all right but had to retire apparently because the men were exhausted from lack of water. We even held Gaza for a time. The net result was that we retired to our starting point after losing much more heavily than the Turks in men and material.[39]

The British losses were quite heavy – 3,967, of which 523 were killed, 2,932 wounded (the majority of them lightly), and 512 missing in action. Another 246 British troops, wounded and unwounded, were taken prisoner by the Turks. The Turkish defenders had about 2,500 casualties, among them 300 dead.[40]

According to the battle plan, ADSs were established by the mobile sections of the field ambulances affiliated to the brigades. ADSs were also established by the 53rd Division and the Imperial Camel Corps Brigade. MDSs were located by the 53rd and 54th Divisions at Deir el Belah and by the 52nd Division at Khan Yunis. A Motor Ambulance Convoy, under the responsibility of DDMS Eastern Force, evacuated casualties from the ADSs of the 53rd Division to MDSs and further to the CCS, which was located at Khan Yunis by the DMS.[41]

The actual process of medical evacuation was very tedious. About 1,282 casualties remained at the ADSs until the dawn of 28 March. There were several attempts by the DDMS and the DMS to influence and improve the professional treatment at the crucial point of the CCSs.

> Colonel H. Wade, of the Scottish Horse Mounted Brigade Field Ambulance, was consequently directed by the DMS, Surgeon General J.H. Maher, to report as consulting surgeon to the DDMS in the field. He assisted the staffs of Nos. 54 and 53 CCS's and further assistance was obtained from the 52nd (Lowland) division, in which there were several surgical specialists.[…] The advanced CCS possessed accommodation for 400 patients only. The number received were much in excess of this and many cases were consequently left on their stretchers in the open, an ample supply of blankets being available for them. These patients were more comfortable and slept better in the open air than those accommodated under canvas.[42]

The agony of the wounded soldiers, together with the problems of the medical services, are reflected through the eyes of Dr. J.J. Abraham, commander of the 24th Stationary Hospital at Qantara:

> As is inevitable in a defeat, the sick and the wounded came piling back. The Field Ambulances cleared them to the 26 CCS and the 2nd Australian Stationary Hospital, both of which were at El Arish; and they sent most of the sick and wounded back to us at the 24th Stationary Hospital, Kantara, by hospital train and in the open trucks of the supply trains. It was a bad show. We never knew how many were killed, but there were 2480 wounded, 1930 of whom passed through our hands at Kantara between March 27th and April 2nd.[43]

Captain P.C. Duncan, of the 2nd/4th Queen's Own Battalion, the 53rd Division, who was wounded on the first day of the battle, left the following report:

> A shrapnel shell burst about a foot from my head, causing the putting out of action of my left eye and driving three shrapnel bullets through my left shoulder and down into dangerous

> proximity of my heart and lungs. [...] I was moved immediately to El Arish where there was a casualty clearing station. This consisted of a number of white marquees with red crosses to warn the Turks to keep off. It was decided that an immediate removal of the shrapnel bullets was vital, possibly even essential, to save my life. Accordingly I was taken to the theatre tent and introduced to the little surgeon who was to carry out the operation on me. I don't think he was English, he had a little beard and indulged in the un-English practice of saying to me 'You'll be lucky if you're alive tomorrow.' The proceeding had got as far as my being told that all anaesthetics were missing, and that the best they could do to cope with the obvious agony which the surgery would involve, was to give me a bottle of Jonny[!] Walker Whisky which was only half full. Part of the other half I had seen (which I wouldn't have seen had there been anaesthesia) poured down the throat of my bearded surgeon.
>
> Then came calamity. Apparently disregarding the Geneva convention a Taube flew over the hospital and neatly dropped a bomb right on top of the surgeon narrowly missing me, but admittedly providing two or three extra wounds. I was whisked away after about an hour of near panic, and for twenty four hours left to survive if I could without any attention.[44]

This was not the only recorded event of deliberate air attacks on well marked hospitals by German airplanes:

> The Taubes are playing hell of nights, dropping bombs all among the big camps. Our hospitals should be completely isolated from the fighting camps. Forty bombs were dropped on a big hospital in Belah. Two Tommy doctors were operating on a man for appendicitis; the bombs were crashing all around them, the concussions rattling their instruments; they worked steadily on and finished the operation successfully.[45]

There were other cases in which enemy airplanes attacked hospitals, though well marked. At least in some of the cases the pilots tried to explain the motives behind their act. A medical officer reported:

> Fritz dropped a message in the morning saying that he had bombed our hospitals as a reprisal for our shelling a mosque in Gaza and for bombing a convoy of his wounded. As a matter of fact, the mosque contained an enormous ammunition dump, which we saw subsequently, after the fall of Gaza, six months later.
>
> It was said that the convoy of wounded, having no distinctive marks on its wagons, was mistaken for a transport column. Fritz also added in his message that he would bomb the hospitals again at 8 p.m. on the same day. It was a moonlight night and he kept his promise but this time only causing about thirteen casualties.[46]

In other cases hospitals were attacked due to what seemed to be British negligence: 'Turkish Airmen used to drop messages asking us kindly to move our hospitals lest they should be hit by bombs intended for the dumps. Presumably out of pure cussedness the hospitals stayed where they were; and inevitably they were bombed. Then they moved.'[47]

The Turks did not waste time after the battle of Gaza, which in few days became a well fortified stronghold. Despite this, the War Cabinet urged General Murray to advance into Palestine and capture Jerusalem. It seemed very important strategically after the great advance of the British Expeditionary Force in Mesopotamia and the taking of Baghdad by General Maude on 11 March. The result was that General Murray, though reluctant, decided to attack Gaza again shortly.

In anticipation of the Second Battle of Gaza, he decided upon the use of gas shells in order to secure a victory this time. Those to be used were CBR shells which consisted of equal parts of the lethal substance phosgene and chloride of arsenic. General Murray had already considered employing gas shells during the First Battle of Gaza. However, this was not done for two main reasons: Murray's inconsistent policy on the use of gas and the fact that these shells had not arrived in Palestine in time. It was understood that the optimal meteorological conditions for the use of gas shells were during the early morning hours. Later on, winds and higher temperatures would cause more readily the dispersion and disintegration of the gas, and it might be without any real effect on the entrenched Turkish troops. Despite this, the main attack on Gaza was planned for the late morning. It meant a significant time gap between the possible effect of the gas shells and the infantry attack.

Eventually, as a compromise between several approaches and Murray's inconsistent policy on the use of gas, only six artillery batteries fired about 1,800 gas shells during the early morning hours of the first day of the Second Battle of Gaza. When the British troops later assaulted the town, they faced very strong resistance; apparently the gas shells did not have any effect on the defenders. Though there were rumours that Turkish soldiers were actually affected by these shells, there was no real data supporting them.[48]

The DMS tried to study most of the lessons of the First Battle of Gaza. He realized that one of the main problems was lack of coordination among medical units involved in the process of medical evacuation. He therefore decided that while the mobile sections of the field ambulances would follow the brigades in order to establish ADSs, all motor ambulances would be concentrated under the command and control of the DDMS Desert Column.[49] This should contribute to the organization of evacuation of casualties, as the DDMS might see the general picture of the battlefield and where support could be needed. In addition, special traffic routes were allotted solely for evacuation of casualties.

Prior to the British assault, several surgeons were sent from Egypt to assist the staff of the frontline CCS. However, some of them could not function in an optimal way due to lack of surgical equipment.[50]

The Second Battle of Gaza was launched on 17 April 1917 and lasted for four days. The outcome was as in the first round: the defenders managed to halt the British troops who, eventually, withdrew from the town. However, the toll this time was much higher. The British suffered 6,444 casualties: 509 dead, 4,359 wounded, and 1,576 missing in action. 3,118 battle casualties were evacuated from the front line and treated at the various medical echelons from 16 to 21 April. The Turkish losses were much lighter – 2,013.[51]

Dr J.J. Abraham, commander of the 24th Stationary Hospital at Kantara, noted in his published diary:

> It started on April 17th and ended in complete failure on the 19th. Six thousand five hundred sick and wounded men came down the line, most of them to Kantara, where we were the only hospital able to receive them, to treat them and evacuate them to Egypt. [...] The more serious cases came in the two hospital trains. The lighter cases came in the open trucks of the supply trains. [...] The journey started in the morning in hot sunshine, and ended at Kantara generally about midnight, when we took them in by the light of flare lamps. By then it was very cold – the desert air at night can be very chilly – and we found to our horror that a number of them were dead, cold and frozen because the blankets and tarpaulins with which they had been issued had been commandeered en route by an ordnance officer short of stores who thought they did not need blankets and tarpaulins in hot, open trucks. It was a stupid, unimaginative thing to do. We raised hell and it did not happen again.[52]

Did the mounted troops really capture parts of Gaza before they were forced to retreat for various reasons? Dr Abraham had a very interesting medical observation concerning this question:

> Our cavalry got into the streets. And then water and ammunition began to fail. There was some bad intercom staff work and we withdrew. I can now disclose a curious medical fact. Mounted troops actually got into Gaza, and, in emulating Samson, three of them got gonorrhoea. As there was no chance of acquiring this in the desert and as none of them had been on leave in Egypt, we were satisfied they really had been inside Gaza.[53]

One of the medical lessons learnt from the two battles of Gaza was that two adjacent hospitals working in coordination with each other were more efficient than two hospitals operating each on its own. The first of such 'pairs' was established at Qantara, where No. 44 Stationary Hospital joined No. 24 Stationary Hospital. The DMS located the next pair of hospitals – Stationary Hospitals Nos. 43 and 45 – at Masaid, along the evacuation route from Palestine to Egypt.[54]

As a result of the second failure at Gaza, General Dobell was sent back to England. In his fourth despatch, dated 28 June 1917, General Murray tried to explain the dismissal of General Dobell on medical grounds:

> In the meantime it became apparent to me that General Dobell, who had suffered some weeks previously from a severe touch of the sun, was no longer in a fit state of health to bear the strain of further operations in the coming heat of summer. To my great regret, therefore, I felt it my duty to relieve him of his command.[55]

General Chetwode succeeded Dobell as commander of the Eastern Force; Major General Harry Chauvel replaced Chetwode as commander of the Desert Column, and Brig. Gen. Edward W.C. Chaytor, commander of the New Zealand Mounted Rifles Brigade, succeeded Chauvel at the command of the ANZAC Mounted Division.

After the second defeat at Gaza, the policy of the War Cabinet also changed and the mission of the EEF ceased to be the taking of Jerusalem but rather 'to take every favourable opportunity of defeating the Turkish forces opposed to him, and to follow up any success gained with all the means at his disposal, with the object of driving the Turks from Palestine, as and when this became practicable.'[56] As an outcome of the change of policy, the War Cabinet also decided to reinforce the EEF with an infantry division. The one selected was the 60th (London) Division, then in Salonika, which had seen battle on the Western Front before it was sent to Macedonia. The division, commanded by Maj. Gen. Edward S. Bulfin, began to join the EEF on 14 June.[57]

As a result of British international political agreements, three French battalions arrived in Palestine on 25 May 1917 in order to join the forces of the EEF. The French troops formed the French Palestine and Syria Detachment (Détachement Français de Palestine et Syrie – DFPS). The detachment also included cavalry, artillery, and medical units. It was commanded by Colonel P. de Piepape, who would lead this unit throughout the Palestine campaigns. On 13 June 1917 the EEF was also joined by a small Italian detachment numbering about 500 troops commanded by Lt-Col. Cav. F. D'Agostino.[58]

On 11 June 1917 General Archibald Murray received a telegram informing him that the War Cabinet 'considered it desirable to make a change in command' and had decided to appoint General Sir Edmund Allenby to succeed him.[59]

3

GENERAL ALLENBY: THE MAN AND HIS ATTITUDE TOWARDS MILITARY MEDICINE

'He is, I think, the only commander who has fought in that country who did fully understand the position and the seasonal risk.'

Sir James Barrett, 23 November 1932.

'No general, probably, has ever given fuller assistance and support to his doctors in their measures in combating the risks of disease.'

Archibald P. Wavell, *Allenby: A Study in Greatness* (London: George G. Harrap, 1940), 255–56.

On 23 May 1917 General Sir Edmund H. Allenby, commander of the Third Army in France, was summoned to London for briefing before taking command of the Egyptian Expeditionary Force (EEF).[1] For Allenby, this transfer could be interpreted as a dismissal by the Chief Commander of the British Forces at the Western Front, Sir Douglas Haig. Yet, when he came to London and met Prime Minister David Lloyd George and Chief of the Imperial General Staff (CIGS) General Sir William Robertson, he willingly accepted the new assignment and sailed for Egypt.

'The sea voyage,' according to Sir Basil Liddell-Hart, 'is a turning point in Allenby's career as well as in his reputation both as a Commander and Man.'[2] Liddell-Hart's interpretation goes much further:

> Few famous men have been the object of such extremes of condemnation and admiration within the space of few years as Allenby. [...] Most curious of all was the sharp dividing line drawn by a journey through the Mediterranean in June, 1917. For almost three years in France he had been a target of strong criticism. [...] Yet Allenby in Palestine became as a Chief, [...] by no means a human enigma.[3]

A thorough evaluation and appreciation of Allenby's performance during the Boer War in South Africa, as well as on the Western Front during the Great War, is beyond the scope of this book. Yet, one is unable to appreciate Allenby's leadership, as well as his virtues and vices as they were manifested during his command of the EEF, without relating to his military career prior to the Palestine campaigns.

Allenby began his military career with the Inniskilling Dragoons Regiment in South Africa where he served for several years during three different periods of time, the last being in the Boer War. During that war Allenby distinguished himself several times. In April 1900 he assumed temporary command of the Inniskillings and by January 1901 was given charge of an independent column which he commanded until the end of the war in May 1902. During the Boer War, Allenby was much appreciated by his officers and men.[4]

From August 1902 until October 1905 he was commander of the 5th Lancers, a period during which some of his virtues were noticed:

> Under a brusque manner there was unbound human sympathy. He expected all one could give, but was always ready to help in sickness or in trouble. [...] He had a great grasp for the smallest details of regimental life, and during an inspection nothing escaped him. [...]
>
> He was the most willing and capable teacher. [...] He would shoulder full responsibility for any fault found by higher authority, and had consequently the unfailing loyalty of all ranks.[5]

From 1905 until October 1909 he commanded the 4th Cavalry Brigade, after which, until the commencement of the Great War, Allenby, already a general, was Inspector-General of cavalry and commander of the Cavalry Division. He sailed for France with his division when war broke out on the Western Front. The Cavalry Division participated in various battles, including the British retreat during the Battle of the Somme. It was there, on the modern battlefield characterized by trenches and barbed wire, that the role and real value of cavalry in modern warfare was questioned and criticized. Naturally, the officer commanding the British cavalry and acting as its Inspector-General was identified with it and could not escape this criticism.

Yet, in May 1915, after several months as commander of the 1st Cavalry Division, Allenby was promoted to command the Fifth Cavalry Corps; in October 1915 he was promoted once again, succeeding General Charles C. Monro, commander of the Third Army, who had been sent to the Dardanelles. For more than eighteen months, while several senior commanders in the British Expeditionary Force at the Western Front were relieved of their command and despite his strained personal relations with Sir Douglas Haig, the supreme commander of the BEF, he maintained his position. Haig and Allenby were old peers, having studied together at the Staff College (1896–97) and resenting each other ever since.[6] In the spring of 1917, during the offensive at Arras, General Allenby's performance as an Army commander was not to the liking of Sir Douglas.

At that time, after Murray's second failure before the gates of Gaza, CIGS General Robertson sought a successor to command the British Force in Egypt. The first candidate was General Jan Smuts, a South African. When he turned down the position, Robertson considered General Allenby to be the proper candidate for that command. Only then was he summoned to London.

With the arrival of Allenby in Egypt a new epoch began both in his career and in the history of the EEF. Thus, Liddell-Hart was most probably justified in using the 'sea voyage' as a metaphor for a turning point in Allenby's career. But was the sea voyage also the beginning of the creation of a new and previously unknown Allenby? It was Liddell-Hart himself who had this to say about Allenby: 'He had a unique instinct for surprise and mobility.'[7] In that same essay Liddell-Hart wrote: 'Experience had shown Allenby that even the most difficult maneuver was preferable to butting directly against a blank wall; [in Palestine] he found the right field for his gifts and instincts.'[8]

If these virtues had been known before the Palestine campaigns, and

Palestine was indeed 'the right field for his gifts and instincts,' could then the 'Mediterranean voyage' be considered the borderline between the 'old' and the 'new' Allenby? Or should it be looked upon rather as the opening of a gate of opportunities, previously locked for him? Could it be that the fact that 'the Bull' of the Western Front, who previously had not attracted any admiration, turned out to become one of the most celebrated commanders of the Great War, brilliant and charismatic, interfered with assumptions, theories, and even prejudices?

Was General Allenby really a 'human enigma'? Did Liddell-Hart consider irrelevant the circumstances and problems with which Allenby had to cope on the Western Front, mainly his relations with Sir Douglas Haig?[9] 'What were Allenby's rare qualities that made him a great General? One cannot find them during his early career; he was not distinguished during the first phase of World War I. Most probably the fact that he was independent changed him to the better and extracted from him his great virtues.'[10]

All these questions are very relevant to the issue of military medicine during the Palestine campaigns. As will be shown, General Allenby, as C-in-C of the EEF, was a key figure in establishing a unique attitude towards military medicine. He was deeply involved in the field of preventive medicine, probably more than any other commanding general during the First World War. This interest and involvement could not be noticed at the Western Front, where the health problems of the troops were different.

In any attempt to evaluate Allenby's personality and leadership, one has to bear in mind the important remarks of Matthew Hughes[11] and Jonathan Newell.[12] Both scholars relate to the possibility that since many of the descriptions of General Allenby's performance in France had been written after the Palestine campaigns, they may have been influenced by Allenby's later glorious career.[13] Hughes has raised the problem of the hagiography built around General Allenby the man and around the Palestine campaigns, contributing to the distortion of any objective analysis of the historical facts. Newell has pointed out that there have been very few studies concerning the various aspects of the Palestine campaigns.[14]

The attitude towards General Allenby expressed in these pages is based, first of all, on facts – what he actually achieved in the area of military medicine while serving as C-in-C of the EEF during the Palestine campaigns. The moot question, then, is how he was perceived and appreciated by the people who functioned in the medical services, as well as by soldiers who were treated by them or by others who were witnesses at the scene. Allenby himself did not facilitate the work of future historians: he made no notes of his acts or thoughts, never kept diaries, and destroyed every letter or paper he received.[15] Though intriguing, the value of information found in his letters is quite limited.

Many important facts concerning General Allenby's leadership had been noted before he travelled to Egypt: 'He instilled confidence and respect in all his subordinates, officers and men. [...] He earned complete trust of the men';[16] 'He could bear contradiction';[17] 'He always attracted good people to work with him and to be members of his staff.'[18] General Sir George de S. Barrow, who served under Allenby's command both in France and in Palestine, wrote: 'Allenby was always glad to listen to other opinions and advice, provided this was backed by knowledge and common sense. What angered him was stupidity, negligence and, most of all, disregard to orders.'[19]

While commanding the Third Army on the Western Front, Allenby had great difficulty in submitting to the will of C-in-C Sir Douglas Haig, this for two reasons. The first was his non-relations with the man whom he had known since the days at Staff College, the second being Haig's conduct of the war in France. Yet Allenby was loyal and obedient. He could tolerate heavy losses when he thought they were justified. However, during the spring of 1917, when British losses totalled 126,300 while German losses were 67,000, something was changed in him, as if there was a crack in his absolute loyalty. He realized that Haig's strategy of attack was wrong and futile. It was the worst period in Allenby's command: he was blamed for carrying out a mistaken policy while he was unable to criticize it openly. The personal price he paid was very high: he could no longer control himself.

One of his division commanders who criticized General Allenby quite openly was General John S.M. Shea. As a result, Shea – no doubt a very capable commander – was relieved of his command. However, when Allenby sailed for Egypt he took General Shea with him, as Allenby bore no grudge against Shea, whom he appreciated as both a commander and a man. When General Edward S. Bulfin, commander of the 60th Division was promoted to command the XXI Corps, Allenby appointed General Shea to command the 60th Division. Allenby's confidence in Shea was proven correct, for the latter turned out to be one of the most successful and capable division commanders during the Palestine campaigns.[20]

During the spring of 1917, Allenby's outbursts became more frequent and more 'bullish' than ever. For the troops who did not know him well, his behaviour during that time only justified his nick-name 'The Bull' and unjustly placed him among those commanders who did not care to lose their soldiers.[21]

> During the whole of his command of the Third Army Allenby spent the greater part of most days with the troops, visiting the front line, the HQ of his corps and divisions, or the administrative establishments behind the front. His frequent appearances in the trenches, were a source of considerable anxiety to commanders and to the troops. In the first place he never displayed the least concern for his own safety and was not to be deterred from inspecting any trenches he wished to see because they, or the approaches to them, were being shelled; and, in the second place, Allenby's sudden explosions of temper, if he found anything wrong, were to be dreaded almost as much as an enemy bomb. These unfortunate outbursts, often over some comparatively trivial breach of discipline, did much to destroy the good impression that the sight of the Army commander in the front trenches made, and to confirm the legend that 'the Bull' was merely a bad-tempered, obstinate hot-head, a 'thud-and-blunder' general.[22]

A letter written by one of the troops at that time (17 June 1917) is a typical example of misinterpretation of Allenby's behaviour: 'The Army Commander, Allenby, went to Egypt. He is not popular – no stories of his little ways are in circulation, and he is quite unknown to regimental officers and men. The army calls him "Tin-Hat," its "upper circles" call him "The Bull." '[23] The future Field Marshal A.P. Wavell, Allenby's biographer and admirer, was aware of the problem: 'His harsh manner gave the unfortunate impression of a rough obstinate commander who could only charge blindly forward.'[24]

General Allenby was an original thinker before the Palestine campaigns – his opinion on machine guns, as it had come to the fore during the South African War, was a good example. His artillery plan for the '3rd Ypres Campaign' was so original and innovative that neither Sir Douglas Haig nor his GHQ could accept it. It is not implied here that it was a better plan than others; it only suggests that Allenby was an original thinker, and that this did not happen to him suddenly in Egypt for the first time.

Allenby's period of command of the V Corps, with its heavy losses both in defence and in attack, confirmed for the majority of the army his reputation as 'The Bull,'

> [...] though it was not his policy and heavy losses occurred also in other corps, as he was very loyal to his superiors, he was identified by the troops with the policy of 'drive at all costs.' [...] The characteristics of the real man, his love of nature, and of children, his disregard for danger, his loyalty and modesty, were recognized, as usual, by those who stood in close contact with him.[25]

Few people knew their Bible better and read it more regularly than he did.[26] This intimate knowledge would serve him well during his future campaigns in the Holy Land. His knowledge of Greek was very good.[27] His personal courage was demonstrated many times during his military career. He used to cite his mother who had taught him 'whatsoever thy hand findeth to do, do it with thy might.'[28] General Allenby was a kind person;[29] his attitude towards people was humane, and he was blessed with a good sense of humour.[30] It was a fact that throughout his long military career he seldom punished anybody.[31]

One of the very interesting virtues of Allenby was his love of children. During the fighting in France, when his HQ was located at the same place for quite a long time, he took care of several local children, with two of whom he developed a special relationship. In one case when a child was severely injured, General Allenby came often to visit her at the hospital. When he found that her situation was deteriorating, he called in a senior military surgeon for advice.[32]

It might be inappropriate to compare General Allenby as commander of the EEF with his predecessor, Sir Archibald Murray. Not only were the circumstances under which each of them tried to execute War Office policy different, but that policy itself had been changed.[33] However, it is difficult to find two generals who have been so different, both in their career and in their attitudes towards various issues. While Murray was essentially a staff officer and an administrator, Allenby was a line officer, a commander who rose in the field amongst soldiers. He understood them and earned their respect and loyalty. Allenby's removal of the GHQ from Cairo to Kelab, near the front line, a few days after assuming command of the EEF was not too important from the military point of view. However it was a declaration, loud and clear, and the troops understood it as it meant to be interpreted.

Comparison with Murray is important only because General Murray and his various military and administrative acts were part of the background into which Allenby was introduced during June 1917. Lt-Col. J.J. Abraham, a distinguished London surgeon who became the ADMS for the Palestine L-of-C during the Palestine campaigns, had a very interesting observation relating to the two EEF commanders:

> When Murray inspected the hospital I took him round the wards. He picked up the temperature sheet of one patient. 'I see,' he said, with a cold sarcastic smile, 'you don't keep your charts very up-to-date. This is the fifteenth of the month. You've charted him to the tenth only.' I looked at the chart he handed me. 'Sorry, sir. It's the tenth day of the disease, not the day of the month,' I answered. He made no further comment, but he did not apologise. That's why he failed to get the devotion from his Army that Allenby obtained so easily. [...]
>
> In June, 1917, we learnt that Sir Archibald Murray had been recalled home and was being succeeded by General Sir Edmund Allenby. None of us was surprised. Murray was essentially an office wallah, in contradiction to Allenby, who was a front line soldier. It was Murray's foresight and imagination that was responsible for the railway across the desert, and the magnificent idea of carrying the waters of the Nile from Egypt to Palestine. He bridged the desert. But in Cairo he lost touch with his fighting troops, and to that was due his failure as a Commander-in-Chief. Allenby reaped where Murray sowed, and, like the great man he was, he acknowledged this fully in his dispatch in June, 1919.[34]

The influence of General Allenby on morale can never be over-emphasized in considering this campaign. It is the testimony of the most critical and responsible observers that he restored the old personal relationship between leader and troops which was one of the finest traditions of the British Army in the past and one of the keys to its success. He was constantly up and down his line, so that there can have been few commanders in modern warfare who were so well known to their troops. All ranks gave him their confidence, and to a force of many nationalities his character and temperament were of inestimable value.

By now it should be obvious, that all the qualities found in Allenby as commander of the EEF had already been an essential part of his character prior to his landing in Egypt. Thus, the 'sea voyage' was certainly a turning point in Allenby's career, but in no way was a new man born on deck.

Filled with confidence, energy, and conviction, General Allenby sailed for Egypt. In no time 'The Bull' became 'The Chief,' though the old bull awoke from time to time. His appearance influenced all troops: 'He was known as "the Bull" amongst us all and no Commander inspired his troops with greater confidence than he. With his arrival a kind of fresh vitality appeared amongst us.'[35]

It is very interesting to read General Harry Chauvel's letter dated 8 December 1917. This was a genuine observation, written before the future successes in the Palestine campaigns. As such, it is not suspect of being part of the later hagiographic attitude towards Allenby.

> I like him immensely and he appeals to my Anzacs tremendously. He is just the kind of man we wanted here. [...] The great thing is he gets about amongst the troops, looks in at hospitals, [...] has a cheery word for the wounded and does not have a fit if he is not saluted, all of which appeals to the Australians and I think to the other troops also.[36]

Another eye-witness testified: 'All have entire confidence in him and our cause is safe in his hands; he will take care to have everything ready, and he will not move until it is so.'[37]

Even T.E. Lawrence, who was known for his original views and maverick attitudes towards most issues and people, was deeply impressed: 'Allenby, gigantic and red and merry, fit representative of the Power which had thrown a girdle of humour and strong dealing round the world. [...] I might let my

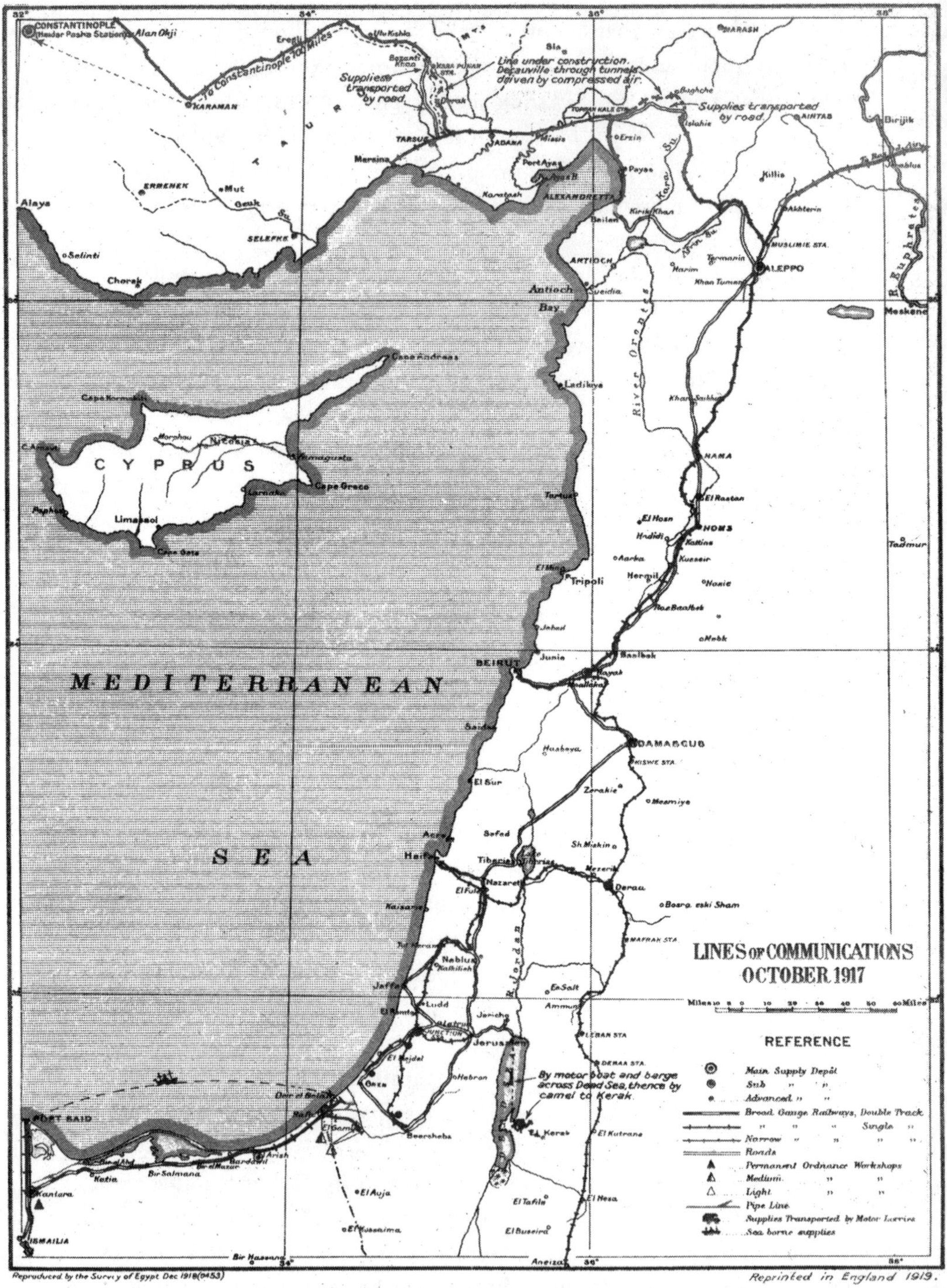

Reproduced by the Survey of Egypt Dec 1918 (9453)

Reprinted in England 1919.

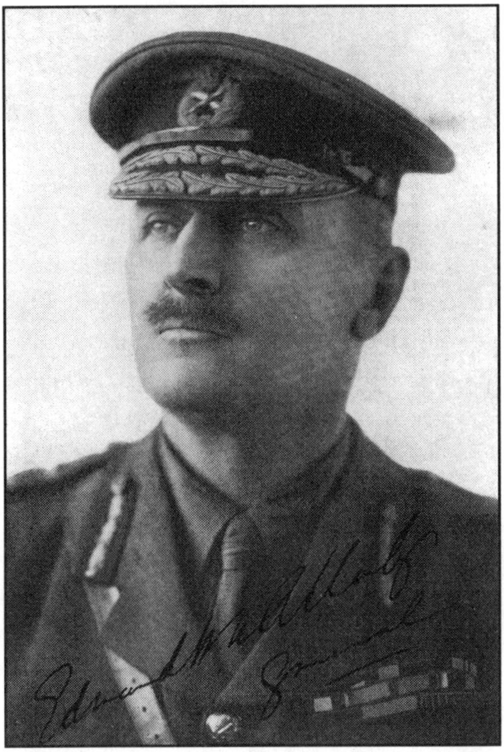

General E.H.H. Allenby

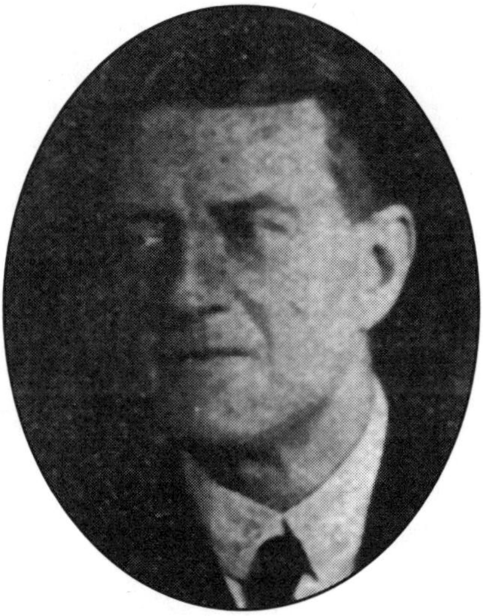

Surgeon General
Sir Richard H. Luce

limbs relax in this dreamlike confidence and decision and Kindness which were Allenby.'[38]

General Allenby was unique in his attitude towards military medicine in general and towards prevention of diseases and medical personnel in particular. His interest in the diseases of Palestine was part of his general interest in anything concerning the area where the future campaign would be fought. However, his interest in science, in general, and medicine, in particular, went far beyond his specific military interest.[39]

While it was the duty of every commander to visit his sick and wounded soldiers at the various hospitals, it seemed that for General Allenby it was more a privilege than a burden. Some even thought that his deep interest in the medical work betrayed an anxious desire for the welfare and health of the men:

> He spent a long time in the ward and insisted on talking to us all and enquiring how we came to be there, what units we came from and in what particular section of the line we had been serving. He gave the appearance, and I am sure it was perfectly genuine, of really being interested in our various experiences. He was a great soldier and a great man, and I think that we were all of us proud to have served under his command.[40]

Already as a commander in France General Allenby extended his help to the medical system:

> Especially was he careful with regard to the medical arrangements; and when, as frequently happened, there were conflicting claims between the ordnance, supply, and medical services for the use of a site or building, Allenby insisted always that the safety and comfort of the sick and wounded should be the first consideration. He issued strict orders that no ammunition depot or similar military store which might invite enemy shelling or bombing was ever to be within near range of a hospital or a casualty clearing station. His care for the sick and wounded was shown outside rather than inside the hospitals, and was known to the medical staff rather than to the troops.[41]

Lt-Col. Sir James Barrett, a medical consultant with the EEF, wrote the following appreciation of Allenby:

> I found that I was dealing with a man with scientific instincts; courteous, considerate, and appreciative of the service the Medical Staff could render. He saw clearly that with a slack Medical Service, military operations might become impossible. He never interfered in detail but supported the Army Medical Service thoroughly, finding out where he could repose confidence.[42]

During his first visit to the Palestine front, General Allenby spent some time at medical units. His visit demonstrated both his keen interest in the subject and also his attitude towards the issue of medicine in the military context. [43]

Allenby's main concern was in the field of preventive medicine; his attitude and he himself were much appreciated by key figures in the medical services:

> From a medical point of view the most interesting point in his conduct of the Palestine campaign was his policy with regard to the malaria question.
>
> He is, I think, the only commander who has fought in that country, who did fully understand the position and the seasonal risk.
>
> To me personally Allenby during the campaign and after wards, was always kindness itself and though one could not but feel him to be a distinctly formidable person, one never had any anxiety or hesitancy in putting suggestion to him because one felt sure of a sympathetic hearing and a wise decision [44]

What were the possible roots of General Allenby's attitude towards military medicine?

It would be difficult to answer this question. It might be assumed that it did not stem from his military experience, more or less shared by most of his peers. Nor could it be traced to the education he had received at home. Most probably it originated in his natural kindness and general humanistic attitude.

While commanding the EEF, was Allenby aware of the situation on other fronts and the impact of health problems on the performance of British troops there? The Dardanelles Committee had finished its work before Allenby assumed command of the EEF. Many units which had fought at Gallipoli were now part of the EEF. Yet, there was no mention in Allenby's letters or other people's memoirs concerning this issue. To the best of our knowledge, Allenby never specifically mentioned health problems during the campaign in the Dardanelles.

Allenby was also well aware of the campaign in Mesopotamia, which he mentioned in a letter to the CIGS.[45] General Chetwode also related to that campaign during the planning of the attack on Beersheba.[46] However, no mention was made of the Mesopotamia Commission, the capture of the 6th Division by the Turks, and even not of General Maude's death – probably due to cholera – after the capture of Baghdad only a few months earlier.

General Allenby should have been familiar with the medical situation on the Macedonian front since many soldiers of the 10th Division who joined the EEF before the third battle of Gaza suffered from malaria. The 10th Division had been transferred to Palestine from Macedonia. Did Allenby know that the British Expeditionary Force on the Macedonian front could not attack the enemy due to the high rate of sickness among the troops, mainly malaria and dysentery? If he knew he never mentioned it. The only reasonable conclusion from these questions may be that Allenby's attitude towards the health of the troops, military medicine, and medical officers was genuinely his own.

A last question – but certainly not the least – concerning Allenby's views on military medicine concerns the death of his only son, Lieutenant Michael Allenby, who was killed in action on 29 July 1917, only a few weeks after his father had sailed for Egypt. Michael Allenby was a graduate of Woolich, where he had taken his course in artillery, and then went to the front. During his short military career he had already been awarded the Military Cross for saving human life on the battlefield.[47] The news reached General Allenby while in the field:

> It was the afternoon of his return from this visit that news came of Michael's death. The chief was utterly bowled over, no one knowing him as 'the bull' would have recognized him as the same man. For a week or two he was a broken man, and though

> he carried on with his work he was a pitiable figure. Dalmeny always a great standby was invaluable at that time, and the Chief told Lady Allenby afterwards that if it hadn't been for Dalmeny, he didn't know how he could have carried on.[48]

After a while Allenby read Dalmeny Rupert Brooke's poem 'The Dead.'[49] Then he wrote:

> War takes the best. He was all that one could desire as a son; and I am proud to have been his father. He never gave Mabel or me one moment of trouble or anxiety. We shall remember him only with love, pride and gratitude. There is not a day in his life I could wish be otherwise than as he lived it. In simplicity, gentleness, cheerfulness and honour, he walked; from his birth until his death. I rejoice in every remembrance of him.[50]

Several days after Jerusalem had fallen to the EEF troops under his command, General Allenby wrote his wife:

> Twenty one years ago we were married. Since then I have had twenty one years of perfect happiness. That happiness has been marred by one great sorrow; but the remembrance of Michael will always be with us, and will be nothing but a joy. The sorrow not to have known him would be far greater than the grief of losing him for a while. For all this happiness, I thank you.[51]

This was a letter very typical of this man who, while the British nation rejoiced in the victories at Gaza and Jerusalem, and even compared them to a successful crusade, remained calm, shy, and quite reserved.

He was a general for whom his family was the cardinal source of his strength and yet he kept his private life far away from the public eye. In a few years Wavell would write: "His temper had mellowed with success; and though he still lived up to his reputation as the Bull, and always remained a very formidable personality, the explosions were perhaps less frequent and his natural kindliness reasserted itself sooner than in France."[52] This unusual, complex, formidable, and knowledgeable general was about to assume command over the EEF and to succeed where others had failed.

4

THE THIRD BATTLE OF GAZA: VICTORY AT LAST

'The Medical Service was able to adapt itself to all the difficulties of the situation, with the result that the evacuation of wounded and sick was carried out with the least possible hardship or discomfort.'

General Sir Edmund H. Allenby, Special Order of the Day, 15 December 1917.

General Allenby did not waste any time. A few days after he disembarked in Egypt, he visited the troops on the Palestine Front. For Allenby, who had seen battles during the South African War and on the Western Front, the Middle Eastern Front was a new and unknown arena. During that first visit, which lasted for five days, the new Commander-in-Chief wanted to get a first-hand impression of the front line, its terrain, and its potential problems. He also intended to meet commanders and soldiers of the various units and to sound out the morale of the troops. At the Eastern Force HQ he was glad to meet its commander, Lt-Gen. Sir Philip Chetwode, a cavalry officer whom he had known and trusted for many years. During the visit Allenby heard a detailed evaluation of the military situation at the front, presented to him by Chetwode and his Chief General Staff Officer Brig.-Gen. Guy P. Dawnay.

General Chetwode emphasized several facts. The enemy was well organized and prepared in its lines of defence. If attacked and unable to hold the line, the Turkish army might retreat in an organized manner to form a new line of defence. This meant, according to Chetwode, that a mere breach of the

Turkish lines would not serve any real military purpose, the main objective being the destruction of the Ottoman Army in Palestine. Gaza, the gate to Palestine on the coast plain, the town that the British had twice failed to capture, had become a fortress. Any attempt to take it again might be more difficult and costly than before. According to Chetwode, Gaza should not be the main objective for the third time. This time it should be the left Turkish flank – Beersheba. The small town of Beersheba was defended by a garrison and the Turks did not consider it a British objective, as it was remote and located beyond a waterless desert. Capturing Beersheba, which had a plentiful water supply, would make possible pursuit of the Turkish forces retreating from the front line. It would also facilitate the attack against the central Turkish defence line. Gaza would be attacked when most of the Turkish line had collapsed and the Turkish army demoralized. General Chetwode explained explicitly the virtues of his plan, mainly the element of surprise and exploitation of the cavalry. He also pointed out the main problems for his plan: lack of water and communications difficulties, both being quite important factors which might have a great impact on the whole scheme.

Apart from the obvious results of the C-in-C's visit, mainly familiarization with the arena and the troops, it brought about two very important results. The first was the immediate impact on the troops: 'General E.H. Allenby took over command of the EEF from General Murray on 28th June, 1917. To the ordinary soldier, who seldom knew what is afoot, the training and the general atmosphere seemed to become much more purposeful.'[1] Remarks made by medical officers were even more enthusiastic:

> He was like a breath of fresh air in a sultry room. He came in like a whirlwind. The first thing he did was to inspect the front line and get to know his officers. The next was to move the GHQ from Cairo to Kelab, just behind the front. [...] His presence in the front line acted like a tonic. The men saw him, 'big bull Allenby,' going round the trenches, talking to junior officers, inspecting the lie of the land. A wave of optimism took the place of the depression that had fallen on us after Gaza II. Confidence in the leadership came back. [2]
>
> His personality and forcefulness, which were made apparent to the troops by his frequent visits to the forward areas, quickly

> produced an astonishing change in the morale of the British troops [3]

The second outcome was that Allenby eventually accepted Chetwode's evaluation as the basis for his plans for a future offensive.

On 12 July 1917 General Allenby wrote a memorandum to General Robertson, the Chief of the Imperial General Staff, in which he explained his view concerning the situation on the Palestine Front. In the memorandum he also requested solutions for several issues which, he believed, were a prerequisite for the capture of southern Palestine.

According to Allenby, the Turkish army in southern Palestine was well organized behind defensive lines and consisted of about five infantry and one cavalry divisions. At least seven infantry and three cavalry divisions were needed to drive the Turks from their positions and reach the Jaffa–Jerusalem line. General Allenby thought he might need more forces if he wished to achieve more than that. He therefore requested reinforcements in infantry units (two divisions), elements of the Air Service, artillery, and signalmen. He also asked for units of engineers, mainly to deal with water and transportation issues. Allenby also specifically requested reinforcement in medical units: two general hospitals, two stationary hospitals, two casualty clearing stations and four sanitary sections.[4]

The C-in-C was promised one division: the 10th Infantry Division, then in Macedonia. It was a well trained and experienced unit which had fought at the Dardanelles. However, many of its men were sick with malaria, as were then most of the troops at that front. It was typical of General Allenby's attitude and leadership that he set out to solve the problem that the 10th Division presented:

> It had suffered much from malaria in the Struma Valley, and the medical authorities advised Allenby that it should have a three months' rest before being used for any operations. Allenby went and inspected the division for himself, and liked its look. He cross-questioned the divisional commander, Longley, who had served under him in France, on the fitness of his men to march and fight; and thereupon rejected the advice of the doctors, and trusted to his own judgment that the division would do its job. His judgment was fully justified by events;

> the division stood up to the hard work of the campaign without undue sickness. Allenby's decision was probably also based on psychology; he knew that to leave an Irish division at rest when fighting was toward was likely to be destructive of its morale and discipline.[5]

This was, most probably, the only time during the Palestine campaigns that General Allenby ignored professional medical opinion and acted according to his gut-feeling.

The denial of another infantry division led to the formation of the 75th Division out of regiments already in Egypt. Thus, the number of infantry divisions was eventually seven, as required. Only several of the requested artillery batteries were approved by the CIGS. Doubling the railway line from Qantara to Palestine was authorized on 21 July, and work started at once. It was expected to greatly improve the ability of transportation to and evacuation from the front line. By the end of October it would reach Bir el Mazar, some seventy miles from Qantara.

Medical units began to arrive during the coming weeks: five new CCSs and one Indian Clearing Hospital joined the two existing CCSs, five Stationary Hospitals were added to the existing three, and four General Hospitals, each of 1,040 beds, were added to the seven already functioning for the EEF in Egypt.

General Allenby informed the CIGS that he would command the force in Egypt and on the Palestine Front himself. This meant that there was no more need of the 'Eastern Force' and its separate HQ. Allenby also intended to reorganize the force. The first step taken was to transfer his GHQ from Cairo to Deir el Belah, near the front. On 12 August the Egypt Expeditionary Force was reorganized in three corps and auxiliary forces, in the following manner:

> The XXth Corps, under the command of Lt. Gen. Sir P. Chetwode, consisted of the 10th , 53rd, 60th, and 74th Divisions, artillery batteries, and support units. The Corps DDMS was Col. Richard H. Luce, formerly the ADMS of the Imperial Yeomanry Division;

> The XXI Corps, under the command of Lt Gen. Sir E.S. Bulfin, consisted of the 52nd, 54th, and 75th Divisions, artillery batteries, and support units. The Corps DDMS was Col. C.J. Macdonald, formerly the DDMS of the Desert Column;
>
> The Desert Mounted Corps, under the command of Lt Gen. Sir Harry Chauvel, consisted of the ANZAC, Australian Mounted, and the Yeomanry Divisions, the Imperial Camel Brigade, artillery batteries, and support units. Its DDMS was Col. R.M. Downes, formerly the ADMS of the ANZAC Division;
>
> The 7th Mounted Brigade, with two regiments, was the EEF HQ reserve;
>
> During the first week of September 1917, a "Composite Force" was formed. It included Imperial Service Indian Troops, the 1st Battalion British West Indies Regiment, and French and Italian contingents. The Force numbered altogether about 3,000 rifles, without any artillery.

The participation of the French and the Italian detachments was the outcome of various political agreements and diplomatic considerations between Britain and her allies made far from the Middle Eastern battlefields. These units would continue to fight as part of the EEF throughout the Palestine campaigns.[6] At that time the EEF included more than 200,000 troops, not including the Egyptian Labour Corps (ELC) which numbered about 60,000 non-combatants.

General Allenby continued to work with the same staff he inherited from his predecessor, with two exceptions: Maj. Gen. Louis J. Bols, who had served as Allenby's chief of staff in France, replaced Maj. Gen. Arthur Linden-Bell as chief of staff. To assist him in his very complicated task in the new arena, Brig. Gen. Guy Dawnay was brought in from the Eastern Force. The other staff officer replaced was the DMS: Col. A.E.C. Keble, the ADMS, Egypt, succeeded Surgeon General John Maher, who had been invalided to England. The ADMS EEF for sanitation was Lt. Col. R. Fowler. On 5 September Lt Col. J. Johnston Abraham was appointed ADMS L-of-C Palestine. His DADMS for sanitation was Capt. J.H. Wood.

On 15 August 1917 General Allenby met his Corps commanders. He informed them of his plans for the future offensive in Palestine, but also dwelt on the various difficulties and impediments which had to be overcome to enable the plan to succeed. Palestine was an underdeveloped country, deficient in roads and water supply. The EEF was at the time, and would be in the future, dependent on lines of communication from Egypt, beyond the Sinai desert. As there were no roads, all supplies beyond railheads had to be transported by camels. This entailed an inherent problem of water, of supplies, and most probably also of medical evacuation to the rear. In the military sense it meant that logistic problems might influence the choice of objectives of the future offensive to an extreme extent.

On the other hand, the Turkish opponent shared the same evaluation of the terrain. Its commanders were aware of the supply difficulties facing a British force attacking from the south, especially the lack of water. They expected the British force to launch its future offensive for the third time against Gaza.

General Allenby's plan, based on Chetwode's evaluation, took into consideration two essential factors: lack of water and the limitations of transportation and evacuation. The water shortage should be solved by creating water resources before the offensive, supplying the forces during the fighting, and capturing Beersheba on the first day of the offensive in order to secure its water wells. The principle behind the plan was surprise, based on secrecy and deception.[7]

Dr W.F. Hume, Director of the Geological Survey of Egypt, studied the water problem in Sinai and Palestine for the EEF. He concluded that in the Gaza-Wadi Ghuzze area, water could be found only at Khan Yunis, where 100,000 gallons were pumped daily, and Beersheba. The water shortage was the result of the huge demand for water by the divisions: a cavalry division needed about 120,000 gallons per day, while an infantry division consumed about 60,000 gallons daily. Already in June, General Allenby was aware of the water problem: 'Our own chief difficulty will be in connection with water supply, owing to the fact that there is apparently no water fit for the troops to drink on any part of the enemy's present line between Gaza and Beersheba.'[8]

The crucial issue of water supply was described quite laconically by the ADMS L-of-C Palestine:

> Our great trouble in the battles of Gaza was keeping the troops supplied with water until they could capture the place. This required about 600,000 gallons a day. [...] Our pipe-line was miles behind, and we could only supply water for twenty-four hours to the men and horses. So it meant a quick victory or failure.[9]

600,000 gallons of water were pumped daily at Qantara, but only 36,500 gallons reached the railhead; the remainder was consumed by the railway, by troops, and by the Egypt Labour Corps workers.

To enable the force to advance on Beersheba and attack it, the water sources at Essani, Khalassa, and Asluj had to be developed for the cavalry and the wells at Malaga and Abu Ghalyum for the infantry divisions. A water pipe would have to be laid to Karm from Shellal and Gamli a day before the offensive.[10] A reservoir of 500,000 gallons of water was created at Wadi Shellal, where a dam was constructed near a ravine with a natural rocky basin. A reservoir of 60,000 gallons was built at Imara.

One of the major problems of supplying water for the troops was the time this entailed. The basic water container was a *fantasse*; made of copper, its capacity was twelve gallons. As every camel carried two *fantasses*, it took a very long time to fill the thousands of them. A device was invented by which 2,000 camel *fantasses*, or 24,000 gallons, could be filled in one hour.[11] 30,000 camels were needed to carry one week's water supply for the EEF.

The main idea was to mount an attack against the Turkish army where it was least expected – Beersheba and the left Turkish flank: the Sheria–Hareira line. Speedy capture of Beersheba and its wells by the Desert Mounted Corps would allow the cavalry to advance and cut the Turkish lines of communication. It would also enable the cavalry divisions to cooperate with the infantry divisions of the XX Corps attacking the Sheria–Hareira line to surround the Turkish Army in that area and destroy it. This attack should commence as soon as possible after the fall of Beersheba.

The role of the XXI Corps was to lure the enemy to Gaza so as to facilitate the offensive of the Desert Mounted Corps and the XX Corps. The plan was that four days before launching the attack against Beersheba, the XXI Corps artillery would begin heavy shelling of Gaza. Two days later the artillery barrage would be joined by bombardment from the sea, but Gaza would be attacked only during the last stage of the offensive. General

Allenby approved the use of gas shells as a part of the artillery plan. It was assumed that bombardment with gas shells would lend force to the plan of deception and lead the enemy to think that the main goal of the offensive was once again Gaza.[12]

THE MEDICAL PLAN

The EEF medical plan for the offensive assumed that most of the casualties were to be expected on the right flank, during the assault against Beersheba and the Sheria–Hareira area. The estimated number of casualties for the offensive was based on one of the formulae used by the RAMC at that time. It assumed that the number of expected cases was ten percent of the attacking force. If the attacking force had been estimated as three-fifths of the whole force, then the number of casualties expected would be 6 percent. Another method used to estimate the number of casualties followed the formula of 10 percent of four-fifths of the entire force, which meant 8 percent of the total Corps.

The XX Corps numbered about 70,000 men. According to the first method of calculation, the number of casualties expected would be 4,200, while if the second method was followed it would be 5,600. The estimated number of casualties in the orders issued for the attack of the XX Corps was 5,000, and medical officers at the various levels were ordered to make all their arrangements for the offensive with that number in mind.[13] In the XXI corps the estimates were based on the assumption that half of the brigades would be simultaneously engaged in battle and that in these brigades about 20 percent of the combatants would be injured.[14]

The ADSs were to serve only as Collecting Posts from which casualties would be evacuated by *cacolet*s or sand carts to the MDSs. It was specified that no operations were to be performed at the Stations level. This was the first time during the Palestine campaigns that Thomas' splint, a simple and efficient device for the initial treatment of thigh and leg fractures, was supplied for general use at the various stations of the field ambulances.[15] It was recommended that every field ambulance open only one MDS, about 3–5 miles behind the firing line. All MDSs were to establish themselves at locations accessible to motor ambulances.

The EEF medical plan called for the operation of two railheads. The first was to be established at Imara Station, about three miles from the

Shellal Junction, where three CCSs (Nos. 35, 65, and 75) and an Egyptian Hospital for Egyptian workers and Turkish wounded or sick prisoners were to be established. The CCSs would be opened and operated as a group to receive casualties of the XX Corps and the Desert Mounted Corps. Another railhead was to be established at Deir el Belah Station. Two CCSs (Nos. 66 and 74) would be set up there to receive casualties of the XXI Corps. Each CCS would be augmented by 100 RAMC personnel from Egypt. Another hospital for prisoners of war would be established at the Deir el Belah railhead as well. At each railhead there would also be an Advanced Medical Stores Depot.

Four hospital trains were to evacuate wounded and sick soldiers from the railheads at Imara and Deir el Belah to El Arish and Qantara. The evacuation would be under the responsibility of the ADMS Palestine L-of-C.[16] Regulation of evacuation from No. 2 Australian Stationary Hospital and No. 26 CCS, both located at El Arish, would be the responsibility of DADMS Palestine L-of-C, while the OC of No. 24 Stationary Hospital at Qantara was responsible for the regulation of further evacuation of casualties to Egypt. Casualties would be transported on deck of the barges 'Niagara' and 'Indiana.' Each barge could carry 50 lying or 200 sitting casualties to the hospital at Port Said, about a three-hour-long voyage along the Suez Canal.

The XX Corps medical plan stipulated that the DDMS would have direct control over four Divisional Immobile Sections of field ambulances. The section of the 60th Division would be set up near Shellal Junction for the initial stage, while those of the 10th, 53rd, and 74th Divisions would be grouped together and opened at Imara, thus augmenting the CCSs there.

All the Corps' motor ambulances would be under the direct control of the DDMS, who would be responsible for the evacuation of casualties from the divisional MDSs to the CCSs at Imara. During the first day of the offensive they would be moved forward according to the situation on the battlefield. Thus, when needed for evacuation of casualties they would not be too far away.

The plan took into consideration the possibility that the mobile sections of the field ambulances would advance with the forces after the capture of Beersheba. To enable them to move, the immobile sections of the 60th Division from Imara would replace them. The immobile sections would be transported to Beersheba by motor ambulances under orders from the DDMS.

The motor ambulances would also transport to Beersheba the sanitary section of the 60th Division when needed there.

The DDMS XX Corps was to operate a Control Bureau, located at Imara Station, near the CCSs, for distribution of casualties brought in by Corps motor ambulances. Motor Ambulance Convoy No. 35, which had arrived from England, would be controlled and deployed by the DDMS XX Corps during the first three days of the offensive.

Wounded prisoners of war would be evacuated to the Egyptian Hospital at Imara until the capture of Beersheba. After that town was taken, they would be evacuated to a hospital in Beersheba itself.

As an outcome of the medical plan, DDMS XX Corps selected the exact place at Imara where the three CCSs and the other medical units would be located. Together with the divisional ADMSs, the DDMS reconnoitered the area to select the sites for the divisional Dressing Stations during the initial phase of the offensive. The decision concerning the exact location of these sites depended mainly on a good route for evacuation of casualties treated at the stations. The routes to be used were marked on special maps of evacuation and the dangerous turnings indicated by signposts erected beforehand. Sanitation instructions were prepared, including a scheme for water chlorination.[17] The ADMS of the Palestine L-of-C realized that his main problem during the days of preparations was the maintenance of secrecy, as:

> [...] nothing gives strategic plans away to an enemy so much as provision for casualties. So my orders were to erect and open three new CCS's, each of 1000 stretcher beds, between dusk and dawn on zero day as close as possible to Beersheba, at a place called Imara. I said to Colonel Keble, the acting D.M.S., that I couldn't do it. It was physically impossible. He said those were Allenby's orders. I would have 600 Egyptian Labour Corps men attached temporarily to each Casualty Clearing Station to help me, and it just had to be done. [...] Two days before zero we moved the three Casualty Clearing Stations with all their equipment to Imara, dumped everything laid out ready for erection on the sand, covered the tents with more sand and waited for the word 'Go'. A few enemy planes came over reconnoitering, but saw nothing. The railway track for three miles behind was covered with sand. We were just a small dump

> in the desert, harmless, innocuous. [...] At sunset on zero night I gave the order and watched the tents of the three Casualty Clearing Stations go up. The men worked all night by the moon. At five a.m. all 3000 beds were up under cover. It was a grand bit of work.[18]

General Chetwode, commander of the XX Corps, took the issue of medical evacuation very seriously: "The Corps Commander was prepared to court martial any one found walking on it, as it is the only possible track for lorries and ambulances, and if it gives out we are done."[19] From another report we learn:

> General Chetwode made a great point of saving the motor ambulances during periods of inactivity as they were limited in number and could not be replaced. They were, therefore, kept concentrated in the charge of a special RASC Officer, under direct control of the DDMS, and only used for serious or urgent cases.[20]

The basic medical plan of the Desert Mounted Corps had to provide solutions for the treatment and evacuation of casualties resulting from a mounted assault on Beersheba. Assuming everything would work according to the plan and the town would be taken by surprise, the number of casualties was expected not to be too high. The mobile sections of the Light Horse Brigades Field Ambulances were to follow the brigades, treat casualties, and hold them till the town was captured. Then they would take them with them to Beersheba, from where they would be further evacuated by motor ambulances of the XX corps directly to Imara.

The medical units of this corps had also to prepare for another possibility: that Beersheba would not be captured as planned during the same day. Such a situation would naturally be the outcome of strong Turkish resistance and might result in a large number of casualties. It also meant that at least some of the mounted units would have to return to their original bases to water their horses before resuming their attack. In such a case they would have no choice but to bear their casualties back with them to Asluj. Evacuation from Asluj to Imara by motor ambulances would take about ten hours, while evacuation by *cacolet* camels might take about twenty-four hours. This

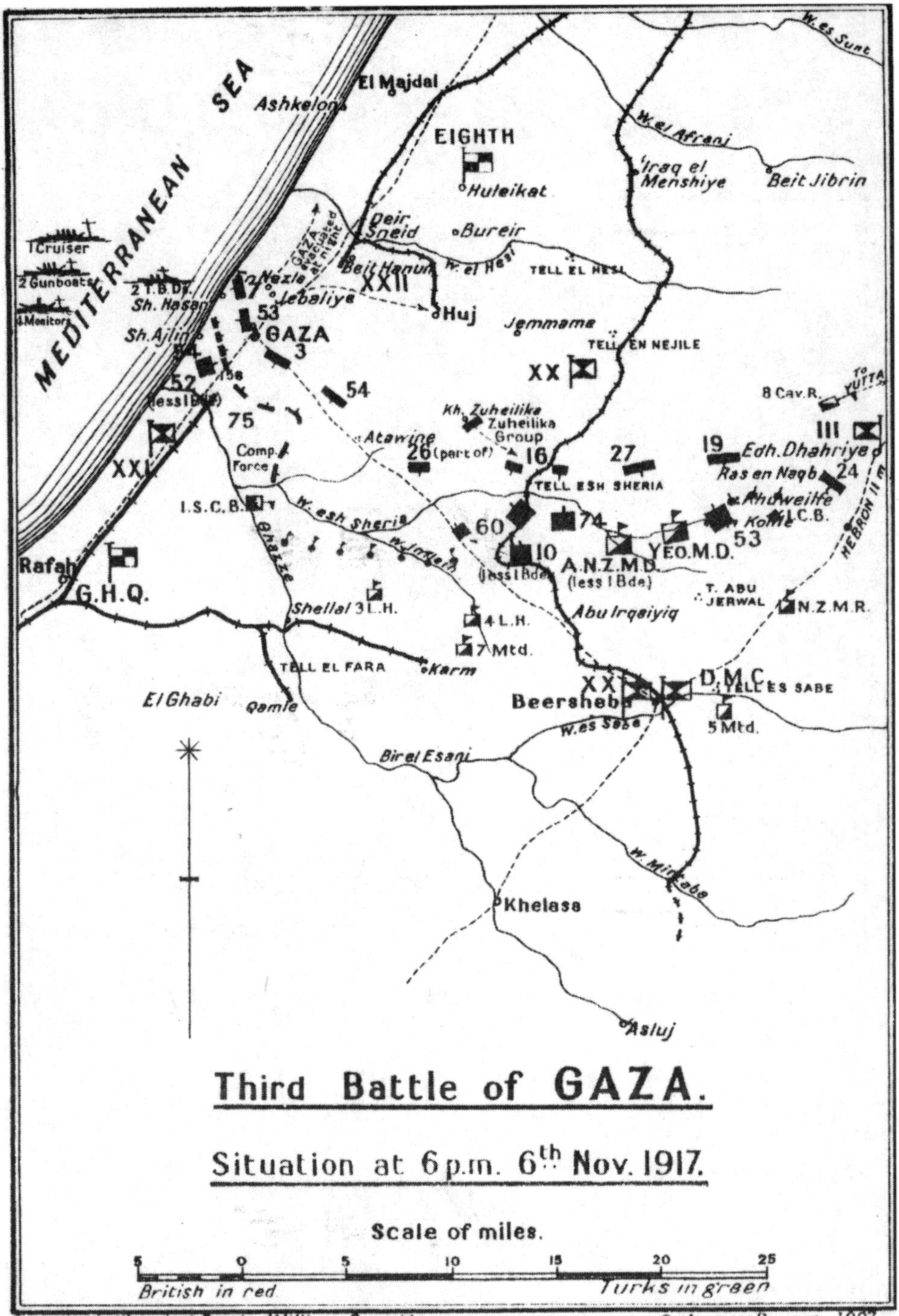

Third Battle of GAZA.

Situation at 6 p.m. 6th Nov. 1917.

Compiled in Historical Section (Military Branch).

Ordnance Survey, 1927.

3000/30.

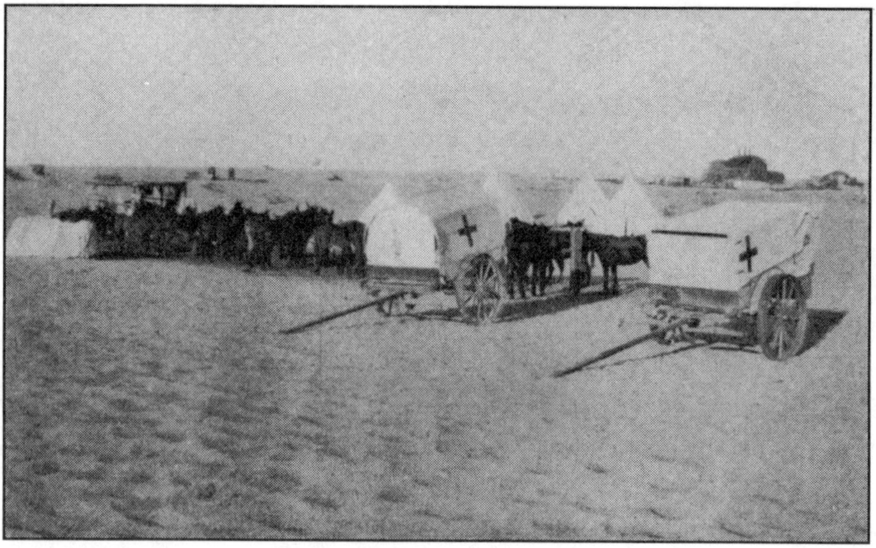

Transport lines of a field ambulance

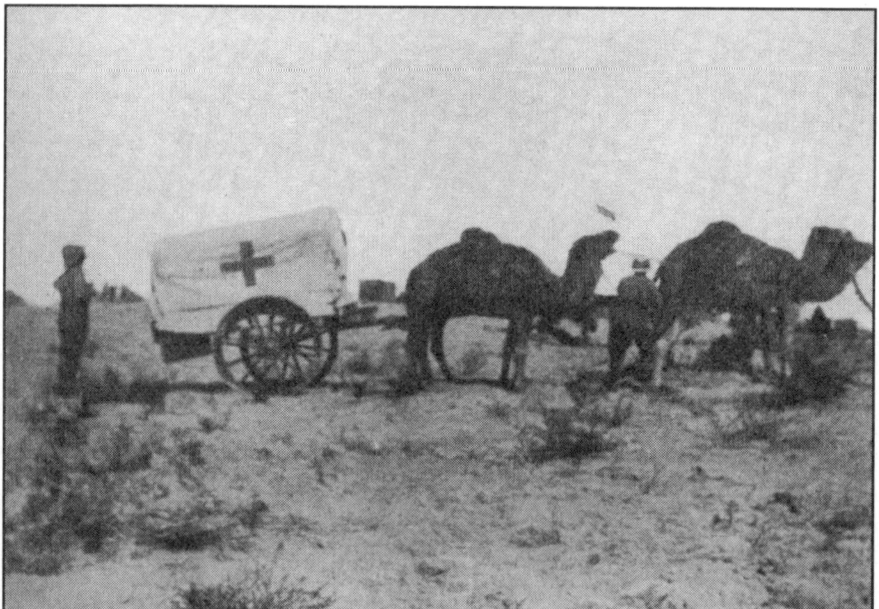

Desert ambulance drawn by four camels

possibility called for special planning and arrangements, as evacuation of casualties from the front line at Beersheba to Imara might endanger the lives of the severely injured, and could be unbearable for all casualties. A special medical problem was posed by those patients who might need an urgent operation; if, indeed, their evacuation would last for so many hours, they had no prospects of being operated on in time.

The medical plan of the Desert Mounted Corps attempted to solve all these problems. The ANZAC Division Main Dressing Station would be located at Rashid Bek, on the route to Beersheba, while the Australian Mounted Division MDS would be located at Bir Asluj. Both would receive orders from the DDMS Desert Mounted Corps. The Advanced Operating Unit would be located at Asluj together with the Australian Mounted Division Main Dressing Station, under command of the DDMS.

The evacuation from the Main Stations to Imara would be executed by means of eighteen heavy motor ambulances from the Motor Ambulance Convoy. Twenty-four of the forty-eight light motor ambulances of the Field Ambulances were retained as a reserve under control of the DDMS so they could be used, when needed, for medical evacuation from the divisions on the battlefield to Asluj or Rashid Bek during the assault. They could also be used, by a decision of the DDMS, to evacuate casualties from Asluj and Rashid Bek to Imara.[21]

While the divisions were advancing towards their destinations, in a detour through arid zones and in complete secrecy, the various medical units moved with them: the mobile sections of the field ambulances with their brigades, the *cacolet* camels behind the divisions.

According to the XXI Corps medical plan the ADSs would be located on the Gaza side of Wadi Ghuzze. They would be sheltered and able to hold 150 casualties each. The distance from the ADSs to the MDSs was planned to be about three miles. Wire roads were prepared for the evacuation of casualties from the ADSs to the MDSs.[22]

In accord with the operations plan, front line medical service was organized in two sectors: the coast sector and the El Mendur sector. The Main Dressing Station for the coast sector would be located at Tel el Nujeid in a sheltered place on the Belah bank of Wadi Ghuzze, near its mouth. Two Main Dressing Stations were to serve the El Mendur sector of operations, both to be established on the Deir el Belah (west) bank of Wadi Ghuzze. Wire roads would connect the Main Dressing Stations to the CCSs at Deir el Belah, the distance between them being about four miles.

A light railway was constructed from Deir el Belah to Tel el Nujeid and thence along the Belah bank of Wadi Ghuzze to El Mendur, its course passing close to all three Main Dressing Stations. Evacuation of casualties from all three Main Dressing Stations to the CCSs at Deir el Belah was to be the responsibility of the DDMS XXI Corps. However, evacuation from the Main Dressing Station at Tel el Nujeid would be supervised personally by the DADMS XXI Corps. Two immobile sections of the Field Ambulances of the 52nd and 54th Divisions were to be opened at Deir el Belah for reception of cholera or suspicious cholera cases. A detachment of soldiers under an officer supported by a sand cart would be allotted to the CCSs at Deir el Belah station to help transfer walking casualties from the trains to the CCSs.

The plan called for the divisional motor ambulances and twenty light (Ford) motor ambulances to be concentrated at Deir el Belah. The DDMS visited the Wadi Ghuzze front and specified the exact locations of the three Main Dressing Stations. Wire roads were prepared and laid on the sand along the routes of evacuation.

A special code was created for the medical units that included specific words for casualties, types of casualties, communications concerning casualties, and their evacuation. All code words relating to casualties began with the letter C.[23]

On 19 October General Allenby assembled the medical personnel of the EEF. He spoke to them about the health of the troops and the medical aspects of the future offensive as he perceived them. Already while in Deir el Belah during his first visit to the front line, Allenby visited medical units at the area, showing his great interest in the health of the troops and in military medicine in general. Colonel Richard H. Luce, who later became DDMS XX Corps, escorted him during that visit:

> He went round our CCS's at Rail-Head and I always remember the sight of him looking down a microscope, while one of our pathologists was trying to demonstrate some Diphtheria bacilli which had just been found to be the cause of those very intractable septic sores from which so many of our troops were then suffering.[24]

THE OFFENSIVE

During the night of 30–31 October the divisions of the Desert Mounted Corps moved swiftly and unnoticed through the unknown terrain from Asluj to the areas east of Beersheba. The full moon assisted them in finding some of the desert paths. They arrived at their area of concentration at Khasim Zanna exactly on time for the coordinated attack on the town from the northeast and east, with the XX Corps attacking from the southwest and west.

At 0555 on 31 October the artillery of the 60th and 74th Divisions began heavy shelling of the Turkish left flank, causing damage to the trenches, casualties among the entrenched troops, and cutting the wire around the trenches. The heavy guns were engaged in counter-artillery fire. The infantry assault began as planned, at 1215, and the line between the Khalassa–Beersheba road and Wadi Saba was captured by dusk. The defences north of the wadi were taken by the Imperial Camel Corps Brigade and two battalions from the 53rd Division.

In the east, the 2nd Australian Light Horse Brigade reached the Beersheba–Hebron road at 1350; a force composed of the New Zealand Mounted Rifles Brigade and the 1st Australian Light Horse Brigade captured well defended Tel Saba after overcoming much resistance. During the late afternoon the ANZAC Division fought its way to Beersheba, which fell to a cavalry charge of the 4th Light Horse Brigade at dusk. The capture of Beersheba was so swift that most of the water wells were seized before they could be sabotaged by the retreating Turkish force. The town was found to be in a terrible state of hygiene. During the night of 31 October–1 November, the Sanitary Section of the 60th Division began its work of disinfection and burial of corpses. It also cooperated with the RE unit in checking the quality of the water in the various wells.[25]

During the last phase of the attack, the Divisional Collecting Stations were erected by the mobile sections of the field ambulances three miles east of Beersheba. The first of these stations was already located at Khasem Zanna by 1230 and began treating and holding casualties there. The second one arrived at 1900 and took over when the first one was loaded with casualties. All 165 casualties of the Desert Mounted Corps wounded during the attack on Beersheba were kept at the Divisional Collecting Stations until the next day.

On the second day of the offensive, at 0700 on 1 November, the Advanced

Operating Unit of the Australian Mounted Division arrived at Beersheba. It took over the Turkish hospital in the town, where most of the casualties were concentrated. About an hour later, the ANZAC Division Dressing Station also arrived there and by 1100 the Motor Ambulance Convoy began the evacuation of casualties to Imara. Throughout the entire operation of the capture of Beersheba the collection and evacuation of casualties operated without any special problems, exactly according to plan.

The concept of the Australian Advanced Operating Unit had been developed during the Sinai Desert campaigns. It was then that cavalry units were assigned long patrolling missions and on several occasions suffered casualties who needed urgent surgical intervention. This unit was commanded by Col. C.J. Storey and had a permanent staff which did not belong to any other medical unit. Though there were those who criticized this unit for being wasteful of manpower, its value and importance in the military scenario of mobile warfare was generally understood. Though this surgical unit worked efficiently while treating casualties at the Second Battle of Gaza, it was employed for the first time under the circumstances of mobile warfare during the capture of Beersheba:

> The surgical car that formed part of the equipment of the operating unit was drawn up adjacent to the window of the room that was improvised as the emergency operating theatre. The necessary sterile warm and cold lotions were already prepared ready for use and the electric cables from the storage batteries of the CAV lighting set on the car were laid into the room and an electric light supplied from this source was suspended over the operating table.
>
> For several days this theatre was used continuously for operating on abdominal cases and other seriously wounded. The car outside was used as a sterilizing and preparing room for the theatre and from it was also obtained a constant supply of electric light which rendered operating much easier and safer for the surgeon and patient alike.
>
> […] The surgical experience gained during these operations confirmed the opinion formed of the value of the unit, consisting of several surgeons experienced in the performance

> of major surgical operations, being immediately available for the treatment of serious cases. It also demonstrated the fact that the equipment required for the performance of such operations was not necessarily either bulky or elaborate, and that a unit of operating surgeons could co-operate advantageously with the various FA's to whose personnel they were attached and whose patients they were treating.[26]

Most of the casualties during the attack of the XX Corps were caused by shrapnel and machine-gun fire while the troops were approaching the enemy's trenches. During this first day of the offensive, the XX corps sustained 1,146 casualties: 136 dead and 1,010 wounded. A high percentage of walking casualties was noted. They were treated at the various stations and evacuated to Imara according to the medical plan.

On several occasions medical units, though well marked by a red cross on a white background, were attacked by enemy airplanes:

> At 6 a.m. on the 1st of November two enemy aircraft descending to 1200 feet bombarded the area occupied by the N.Z.M.R. F.A. still open for wounded, and although red cross flags were prominently displayed, and there were no fighting troops within two miles, yet the aircraft, after expending their bombs, sprayed encampment with machine-gun fire; it seemed deliberately. Bullets and bomb fragments penetrated the tents and bivouacs, tore even the red cross flags, but, by strange providence, the only casualties were one wounded again hit, and one mule killed.[27]

During 1 November, the 53rd Division and the Imperial Camel Corps Brigade advanced to the area of Khuweilfe, north of Beersheba. Khuweilfe was a high hill controlling the whole area north of Beersheba, which also contained several water wells. The 53rd was the only division that retained twenty-one ambulances, as it was scheduled to undertake an independent action. The other divisions had only six ambulances, the rest forming an ambulance park under the DDMS. The Immobile Sections of the Field Ambulances of the 60th and the 74th Divisions were sent to Beersheba to help treat British and Turkish casualties there. On 2 November a Turkish force of more than two divisions counter-attacked the British force at Tel Khuweilfe. The 53rd Division, the 7th Mounted Brigade, and the 1st Australian Light Horse Brigade took part in the battle.

On that same day the Immobile Sections of the XX Corps divisions took over the Turkish hospital at Beersheba from the Australian Mounted Division Receiving Station and the latter moved and continued its work at the Town Hall. Both medical bodies were later busy in treating casualties arriving in Beersheba from Tel Khuweilfe. Beersheba was bombed by enemy airplanes several times, during which some of the medical units were hit.[28] However, neither the medical work nor the process of evacuation of casualties were affected, efforts that were reflected in the diary of a medical officer in the field: 'Our wounded were evacuated from the Collecting Station on the Hebron Road to the Australian Mounted Division Receiving Station in the German Hospital at Beersheba, whence they were conveyed by motor-ambulance to Karm and subsequently to railhead.'[29]

In the meantime, the troops, mainly the cavalry divisions, began to suffer from lack of water. There was a twofold reason for this. First, the Beersheba wells did not supply the expected quantity of water; secondly, the first days of November were extremely hot and dry due to a Khamsin, that extreme hot and dry weather which appears in the Near East from time to time. This is how a Khamsin was described by a British soldier participating in the campaign:

> There was the Khamsin, the 'Breath of the desert' which blew for two or three days at the time in the spring and early summer and which brought sand and dust from the southern deserts. During the Khamsin, the air is like a hot blast from an oven; the driven sand stings; visibility is sometimes reduced to a few yards by flying dust. The heat persists night and day and the whole effect is enervating. But it kills the flies.[30]

As a result, the Australian Mounted Division had to remain at Beersheba and served as a reserve unit. Only the ANZAC Division was able to advance northward to Abu Jerwal, in order to cut the Turkish line of communication at the Beersheba–Hebron road. The 2nd Australian Light Horse Brigade and the 7th Mounted Brigade advanced on the Beersheba–Hebron road and the Khuweilfe area, where they encountered stiff opposition. The 10th Division of the XX Corps took Abu Irgeig, but no further advance was possible due to lack of water.

In the XXI Corps sector, during the night of 2–3 November the 156th Brigade captured 'Umbrella Hill' and at dawn of 3 November the whole front line system of fortifications was taken rapidly by a force of two brigades assisted by six tanks. During the afternoon the British forces successfully repulsed three Turkish local counter-attacks. At the same time, the enemy diverted several reserve forces to the Khuweilfe area, most probably as a result of their evaluation that the Turkish forces in the Sheria–Hareira area might be outflanked by the British. Another possibility was that the advance of a small special British force in the direction of Hebron could not be ignored. That special detachment, 'The Newcombe Force,' composed mainly of trained Arab troops under the command of Lt-Col. Stuart E. Newcombe, R.E., was believed by the Turkish intelligence to be much stronger than it really was. The attraction of enemy forces to Tel Khuweilfe, though so costly to the 53rd Division, contributed much to the success of the XX Corps when its divisions attacked the Turkish army at Kauwaka on 6 November.

On 3 November General Allenby issued the following order to the XX Corps: 'The C-in-C expects Sheria and Nejile to be reached tomorrow.' This order could not be executed since the XX Corps faced severe problems of supplies and water. On the 4th, the commanders of the XX and the Desert Mounted Corps, Generals Chetwode and Chauvel, held a conference after which Chetwode telegraphed Allenby and informed him that the forces would not be able to resume their attack on the Sheria–Hareira line before 6 November. General Allenby agreed to the delay when he realized the serious logistic problems of the various units.

The battle for Tel Khuweilfe was a bitter one which lasted for six days. For the soldiers who fought there, the battle was remembered mainly for the extreme weather conditions and the lack of drinking water:

> The principal engagement in the Third Battle of Gaza was the battle of Khuweilfe, a day's march from Beer Sheba. The battalion was heavily engaged at Khuweilfe and conditions were especially tormenting because water had run out and the thirst engendered in the rocky hills and wadis was more formidable than it is possible to describe. [...] A high percentage of those taking part in this battle had hopelessly swollen lips, and some

> were even driven to drink their own urine which in any event was in short supply.[31]

The battle of Tel Khuweilfe included several attacks and counter-attacks by the opposing forces and heavy casualties were inflicted on both. The 53rd Division bore the lion's share of this battle, its 158th Brigade sustaining 620 casualties during two days, the 6th and 7th of November.

The medical officers of the various combat units treated and evacuated injured soldiers under heavy fire for long hours. An extreme case was that of Capt. John Fox Russell, Medical Officer of the 1/6 Royal Welsh Fusiliers, 158th Brigade, 53rd Division. He had already distinguished himself during the First Battle of Gaza, where 'He showed the greatest courage and skill in collecting wounded men of all regiments, and in dressing them under continuous shellfire.'[32] For his performance in that battle he was awarded the Military Cross Medal. During the battle at Tel Khuweilfe Capt. Fox Russell distinguished himself again when he collected and dressed injured soldiers under heavy fire until he himself was killed. He was awarded the Victoria Cross posthumously,

> For most conspicuous bravery displayed in action until he was killed. Captain Russell repeatedly went out to attend to the wounded under murderous fire from snipers and machine guns, and in many cases where no other means were at hand carried them in himself although almost exhausted. He showed the highest possible degree of valour.

Captain John Fox Russell thus became the only case of an RAMC personnel who was awarded the Victoria Cross during the entire Palestine campaign.

The Turks eventually retreated from Khuweilfe on the evening of 7 November as part of a general retreat of the Ottoman Army. After evaluating the situation, the Turkish commanders decided to withdraw and form a new defence line.

On 6 November the XX Corps resumed its attack on the Sheria–Hareira defence line. During the battle, the 74th Division was fighting quite far from the Beersheba–Gaza road. This created difficulties for evacuation of the casualties from the Division Receiving Station to the Main Dressing Station. The DDMS XX Corps sent a combined immobile section of a field

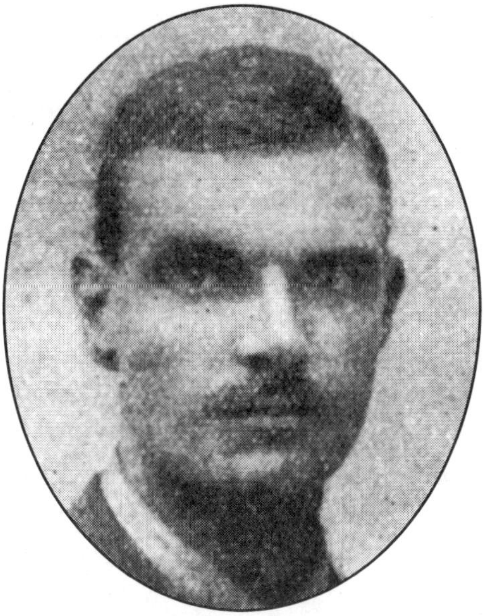

Captain John Fox Russell, V.C., M.C., RAMC

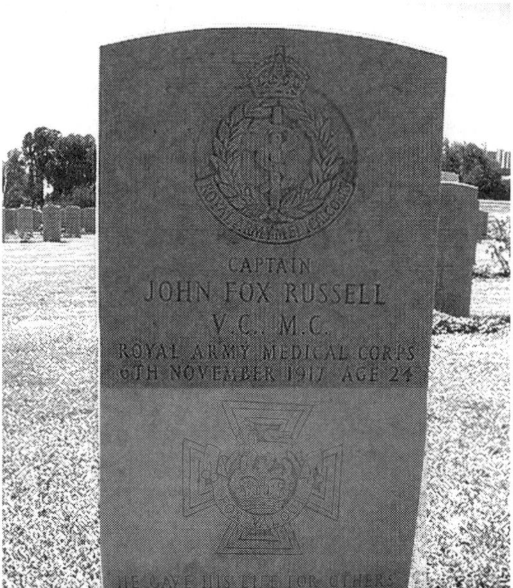

Tomb of Captain John Fox Russell

ambulance to the area from Imara. The casualties of the 74th could then be treated in this new station and evacuated directly to motor ambulances which could reach it. The time thus gained was very important for the casualties, since the previous day the special road to Imara had been heavily damaged due to the heavy traffic, and the process of evacuation before definite treatment had become very tedious.

The continuous bombardment of Gaza demoralized the Turkish troops there. While individuals defected and several units began to withdraw from the town, the fighting of most of the defenders became less resilient. When at 0740 on 7 November the 75th Division took Tel Ali Muntar, one of the key positions of the Gaza defences, it became apparent that the Turks had abandoned Gaza. The town was occupied that same day by several brigades that entered it from various directions. Gaza, the gate to Palestine from the south, previously a symbol of resistance against the British, was found to be in a deplorable condition. On that very day the divisions of the XX Corps also took the Sheria–Hareira line.

During the last phase of the XXI Corps' battle, casualties from the coastal and El Mendur sectors were evacuated by *cacolet* camels and sand carts to the Main Dressing Stations. Four motor ambulances were allotted to each MDS, evacuating lying casualties to the CCSs at Deir el Belah. Walking wounded were evacuated from the MDSs to the CCSs by the light railway. In few special cases motor ambulances were used for direct evacuation from ADSs to the CCSs. Special arrangements were made for the rapid evacuation of urgent cases at night. They were brought by sand carts to the main Gaza road beyond Wadi Ghuzze where a motor ambulance waited and transported them directly to the CCSs at Deir el Belah.

The DDMS XXI Corps, who was at the HQ at Deir el Belah, controlled all these planned and improvised evacuations through a well established communications system, including a motor cyclist near every divisional ADMS. During all these operations the four hospital trains evacuated large numbers of casualties from the CCSs at Imara and from Deir el Belah to hospitals at El Arish and Qantara. The evacuation by hospital trains began as early as 1 November when Hospital Train No. 48 evacuated 397 casualties from Imara, 149 of them being stretcher cases. During November Hospital Train No. 50 evacuated 9,150 casualties from the Palestine front to El Arish and Qantara.[33]

During the operations between 31 October and 9 November, including the capture of Beersheba and Gaza and the destruction of the Turkish front line, the EEF suffered 13,099 casualties. The XX Corps sustained 5,484 casualties: 932 dead, 4,444 wounded, and 108 missing in action. The XXI Corps sustained 2,696 casualties: 361 dead, 1,963 wounded, and 372 missing. The Desert Mounted Corps sustained 4,919 casualties, only a few of them during the battle of Beersheba – 53 dead and 144 wounded, the rest being inflicted on the Corps during the advance northwards.[34]

All these casualties were treated and evacuated by the EEF medical services during less than three weeks. When compared to the number of casualties sustained by the British Expeditionary Force on the Western Front during the various offensives at that time, this was a minor figure. However, relating this number of casualties to the total number of troops in the EEF, it becomes quite a high figure, for about 17.5 percent of the force was evacuated. The actual figures, most probably, were much higher, as this number included only some of the sick soldiers who were evacuated to hospitals. Several thousand sick and wounded Turkish prisoners of war were also treated and evacuated by the medical services.

Hundreds of battle casualties underwent operations in various medical units: the Advanced Operating Australian Unit, various CCSs, and hospitals. The Sanitary Sections coped with all possible sources of contagious diseases, and no outbreaks were noted. All this was done according to meticulous planning and precise execution of the plans. If the victory during the Third Battle of Gaza is attributed to ingenuity in planning and vigour in execution, the success of military medicine during this campaign has not been a beat inferior to it.

5

THE LONG WAY TO JERUSALEM

'The medical services had also performed admirable work under heavy strain, above all the Field Ambulances of the divisions.'

Cyril Falls, *History of the Great War: Military Operations Egypt & Palestine, from June 1917 to the End of the War*, vol. 1 (London: HMSO, 1930), 264.

The capture of Gaza was not the end of a campaign; rather it was a beginning. Since Gaza had been defined as the 'southern gate to Palestine,' the time had come for the EEF to exploit the advantages of that gate, now wide open. General Allenby's original plan was to push on the cavalry to intercept the retreating Turkish armies and cut their lines of communication and routes of retreat. It had been assumed that the beaten Turkish armies would be disorganized and demoralized, easy prey for the cavalry and the Royal Flying Corps (RFC).

Reality was quite different. Due to lack of water, the mounted divisions could not pursue the retreating enemy in full force. At any given time one of the units had to stop to water the horses, returning to a railhead or a known water source for that same purpose. The Khamsin, that extremely hot and dry weather which may appear in the Near East during the autumn and spring, struck Palestine on 10 November for several days, aggravating the water problem. Due to the nature of the terrain, transport of supplies was difficult and limited. In addition, the Turkish army did not retreat in accordance with British expectations. Though many units were broken, scattered, and disorganized, others made an orderly retreat, using the tactic of strong rearguards which fought the pursuing British regiments, inflicting on them casualties and checking their advance. Thus, although mounted and infantry forces were following the retreating Turkish army, pressing its units northwards and not allowing it to establish new defence lines along the main wadis, this was not done according to a detailed plan.

On 7 November only four battalions of the entire Desert Mounted Corps were ready for the pursuit. They advanced through Ameidat Station without facing real resistance. However, their main problem was still water, and the ANZAC Division was pushing its way towards Tel Nejile and Jemmame where water was expected to be found. At the same time, the 52nd Infantry Division of the XXI Corps marched northward from Gaza and by night reached the northern bank of Wadi Hesi, near its mouth. This prevented the enemy from establishing a new defence line along the closest natural obstacle. The RFC attacked the retreating Turkish forces from the air, dropping bombs and firing at them with machine guns. The airmen also served as a good source of intelligence, reporting the enemy's situation to the advancing ground forces.

At dawn of 8 November the ANZAC Division watered its horses at Jemmame, but its advance towards Bureir was checked by Turkish rearguards using heavy machine guns. The Australian Mounted Division advanced on Huj, as did the 60th Division. All attempts by the mounted brigades to seal off the area north of Wadi Hesi in order to block the retreat of the Turkish units proved unsuccessful, for most of the Turkish forces had already left that area. Only one retreating Turkish column was intercepted near Huj.

The encounter that developed with this enemy column would immediately be remembered as the 'Huj Affair.' It was the first occasion in the Palestine campaigns on which swords were drawn and actually used by mounted troops. Though the enemy was driven from Huj, suffering heavy losses, those of the 5th Mounted Brigade which charged the Turks at Huj were not light either: 26 dead and 40 wounded, many of the casualties being officers. After the 'Huj Affair' the Yeomanry medical officer recorded in his diary:

> We commenced to dress the wounded at once, and found them scattered in all directions. Wounded Turks came crawling in, and one could not help contrasting their clean wounds, caused by our sword-thrusts, with the ghastly wounds sustained by our men from shell fire and saw-bayonet. Part of a Turco-German

> Field Ambulance, which had been unable to escape, was found in a hollow behind the batteries, and their equipment was invaluable to us, as our dressings soon ran out and our Field Ambulance had not yet arrived; the Turkish orderlies were put to work amongst their own men, and the intelligent German sergeants proved quite useful. Our little force after the charge was now scattered and very weak, on account of the heavy losses it had sustained, and one could not help wondering whether the Turkish infantry, who had retired only a short distance, would not counter-attack when they saw that we had no supports. However, the enemy had apparently had enough of it, but one was relieved when the first regiment of the Sixtieth Division joined us; the latter were quickly followed by an infantry Field Ambulance from the same Division, a few of whose bearers had been already on the scene.[1]

That same day, General Allenby decided to push forward the XXI Corps along the coastline. To enable this advance, all the means of transport that had been allotted to the XX Corps before the battles of Beersheba and Sheria were returned to the XXI Corps. The principal problem of the advancing EEF units was then, as it would be during the coming days, lack of supplies and shortage of water.

The advance of the various divisions northwards continued during the next days. When the Khamsin struck the whole country on 10 November, the ANZAC Division had already captured Sdud. On that day, as the 157th Brigade of the 52nd Division marched towards Sdud, its medical teams had to take care of 82 soldiers who were heat exhausted.[2] Later on the 52nd Division established itself at Beit Duras and the 75th Division at Julis. This was the first occasion during the Palestine campaigns on which troops were reported to be suffering from heat stroke. Surprisingly, it was also the last one; this episode was unique, though lack of water among the various units was quite frequent. It seems that the unique circumstances of exhaustion together with a Khamsin contributed to the evolution of this event, the likes of which were well prevented in the future.

While there was no detailed plan for the advance, the medical services continued to operate according to basic principles which guaranteed appropriate medical solutions for the various developing scenarios:

> As the troops advanced, pushing the Turks before them, our medical arrangements were that the Immobile Sections of the Field Ambulances should stop at convenient sites, whilst the Mobile Sections went on with the advancing troops, sending back their casualties to the Immobile Sections. Then, as railhead advanced, we of the L. of C. pushed forward a CCS to take over from the Immobile Sections; and they moved on again to another site behind the advancing army, remaining there, collecting sick and wounded, until we and the railway overtook them once more. [...] There was thus officially a CCS at railhead ready always to receive the sick and wounded, and send them back by ambulance train to the nearest Stationary Hospital, or even at times to the Base.[3]

Next day, 11 November, the 52nd and ANZAC Divisions established themselves on the banks of Wadi Suqreir, seven miles north of Wadi Hesi, depriving the enemy of the opportunity to form there its next possible line of defence. The 60th Division was still at Huj and the Australian Mounted Division at Faluja. According to intelligence, including pilots' reports, the Turkish army was organizing and consolidating its divisions in two main areas: the hills north of Hebron, protecting the southern approach to Jerusalem and the area east of Ramle, and around the Junction Station. RFC airplanes bombed the Junction Station.

Even though at that time Jerusalem was only a remote strategic goal, the Junction Station was a desirable and achievable objective. It was one of the most important railway junctions in Palestine, where the Jerusalem–Jaffa railroad met the railroad to Beersheba and Gaza, leading on to Deir el Belah and Egypt. Capturing the Junction Station meant for the EEF acquisition of important ability to supply the forces advancing towards Jerusalem and Jaffa. To the Turkish army it would mean the loss of a main railroad and of any future flexibility in supplying its units.

Thus, it was expected that the British advance towards the Junction Station would face strong resistance. At that time not only the Turkish prisoners were suffering from health problems such as dysentery and exhaustion.[4] The British troops too, mainly the mounted units, began to show signs of exhaustion and health deterioration. This was clearly recorded in the diary of the Yeomanry Medical Officer:

> (November 11) During the morning a large number of sick men and horses were evacuated. The strain was beginning to tell; we had now been on the move for fourteen days, and the horses had on more than one occasion been forty-eight hours without water and often twenty-four; on many occasions the latter had been equally long without having their saddles off – the men were badly in want of sleep, and many had broken out again with septic sores chiefly on account of their inability to wash or to take off their clothes for the past two weeks. A certain amount of dysentery also began to develop again. However, the advance had got to go on, however great the wastage in men and horseflesh might be.[5]

On 12 November several brigades were engaged in combat with Turkish units at various locations. At Balin, the Turks counter-attacked the advancing British forces and were repulsed with heavy losses, while the British sustained only light casualties. At Burqa, the 156th Brigade of the 52nd Division was fighting against a well organized Turkish rearguard. Though eventually the enemy was driven away, it inflicted quite heavy casualties on the brigade: 92 killed and 322 wounded. Together with the losses of the 75th Division and the 1st Australian Light Horse Brigade, who were also fighting the enemy in adjacent areas that same day, the EEF losses for 12 November were about 500.

While the cavalry divisions were advancing northward, the Advanced Operating Unit of the Australian Mounted Division accompanied them and treated casualties when necessary. Its two main stops on the way to Jerusalem were first at Julis and then at a monastery in Ramle.

During these days the retreating enemy formed a new line of defence from El Qubeibe in the west to Beit Jibrin in the East, held by about 20,000 Turkish troops. The key sector of this defence line was the ridge on which the villages of Maghar and Qatra were situated. This ridge also protected the important Junction Station from the southwest. It was understood that any attempt to take the Junction Station depended on capturing the ridge, including these two villages.

On 13 November the 156th Brigade of the 52nd Division took Qatra from the south, assisted by an assault charge of mounted troops from the north. Simultaneously, the 155th Brigade of the same division together with the 6th Yeomanry Mounted Brigade took Maghar. The enemy put up a firm resistance, and though the Turkish troops were scattered by the end of the day they inflicted more than 600 casualties on the attacking forces, most of them from the 155th Brigade which sustained 100 killed, 506 wounded, and 10 missing. During that same day the 75th Division captured Mesmiye, its losses totalling 506: 63 killed, 414 wounded, and 29 missing. After the fall of Maghar a hospital for wounded and sick Turkish soldiers was established at the local sheikh's house.[6]

Throughout the night of 13–14 November the brigades of the 52nd Division approached the Junction Station, which was eventually occupied at dawn on 14 November. The British troops found there large quantities of supplies and ammunition, as well as guns and machine guns. In addition there was a functioning Turkish Field Hospital; its medical staff – doctors and orderlies – were attending the sick and the wounded who could not be evacuated when the British troops captured the area.[7]

During the attack by the 75th Division on Mesmiye, its MDS was located at Suafir el Gharbiye, and next day it was established at El Qastine. When the 52nd Division advanced towards the Junction Station, its advanced dressing stations were established at Mesmiye and Beshshit, with the divisional main dressing station located at Sdud. The treatment of casualties at these advanced medical echelons did not present any unexpected problem.

The main problem at that time was medical evacuation from the MDSs to the CCSs which were still at Deir el Belah, some thirty miles to the rear. Casualties were evacuated to the CCSs by motor ambulances of the corps, assisted by motor ambulances of the 35th Motor Ambulance Convoy which arrived on 13 November. All available supply and ammunition lorries returning empty from the front also assisted in medical evacuation. All these activities were directed and coordinated by the DDMS XXI Corps.

One could not overestimate the importance of the capture of the Junction Station. That event had divided the retreating Turkish army into two separate bodies: the Eighth Army was retreating to the north, in the direction of Jaffa, while the Seventh Army was making its way to the east, into the Judean hills. It was also the first time since the pursuit had begun that the EEF had unlimited access to water.

The mounted forces continued to press the enemy northwards, the ANZAC Division advancing on Jaffa while the Yeomanry Division approached Ramle and Lydda. At Ayun Kara, six miles south of Jaffa, the New Zealand

Mounted Rifles (NZMR) Brigade fought a superior force of the retreating enemy. Though the brigade won the battle by a charge, the cost of victory was quite high: 44 killed and 81 wounded, 'nearly 18 per cent of casualties amongst the 700 rifles actually engaged, and the proportion of killed to wounded was unusually high.'[8]

The medical services of the NZMR Brigade were fully occupied during the engagement. Already when on its way, the NZMR Field Ambulance was instructed by the ADMS ANZAC Division, Col. D.G. Croll, to open an MDS at El Qubeibe, three miles north of Yibna. It had been a wise decision, for within an hour after the engagement had begun battle casualties were arriving at the MDS. An hour after the battle of Ayun Kara had ended the MDS was congested with all the casualties evacuated hence from the battlefield. All were fed and properly treated when four hours later, upon the orders of the ADMS, the 1st Australian Light Horse Field Ambulance arrived at El Qubeibe and relieved the tent subdivision of the NZMR Field Ambulance. Two hours later, all the casualties were evacuated to Yibna. The NZMR Field Ambulance continued its work by treating about ninety sick troops and several Turkish casualties.[9]

After the battle at Ayun Kara the road to Jaffa was open and that town was entered two days later by the NZMR Brigade without opposition. The ADMS L-of–C ordered CCS No. 77 from Gaza to advance to Jaffa.[10] It would arrive there ten days later. However, the DDMS Desert Mounted Corps on the scene was faced for the first, but not the last, time with the task of organizing medical and sanitation services for the captured town. The official history version of the medical and sanitary action is quite laconic: 'The only civil hospital was French, with a staff of two nurses: this was taken over and organized by the New Zealand Field Ambulance. The cleansing of the town was effectively carried out by the ANZAC Division's sanitary section with the help of gangs of sweepers and six incinerators.'[11] The New Zealanders seem to have seen it quite differently:

> A regiment of N.Z.M.R. had entered Jaffa two days after the action at Ayun Kara. Lieut.-Col. Hand Newton was ordered to proceed there on the 17th for the purpose of taking over the French Hospital, but the buildings were found to be in such an unsavoury condition, due to hurried withdrawal of the Turks, that after Herculean efforts, the small staff of the Tent

> Subdivision – the bearers being still with the Brigade – found it impossible to cleanse the wards satisfactorily. The mattresses were heavily infested with bed bugs, mosquitoes extraordinarily prevalent, and the sanitary offices and the water supply were in a dangerous condition of neglect and disrepair. In fact, as some wit suggested, the hospital seemed to have remained unopened since the retreat of the French Syrian Force from Jaffa on May 27th, 1799, on which day the army surgeon, Desgenettes, indignantly repudiated Napoleon's suggestion that the 60 moribund sick, about to be abandoned, should be granted euthanasia by an overdose of opium. Lieut.-Col.Hand Newton reported to the ADMS that the French hospital was unfit for occupation and on the 20th, General Chaytor, whose headquarters were now in Jaffa, arranged for the Mounted Field Ambulance to take over a portion of the Jewish college as a garrison hospital.[12]

During the morning of 15 November a force from the Yeomanry Mounted Division captured the high hill of Tel Gezer east of Ramle, which controlled the road to Jerusalem. This action enabled the taking of Ramle and Lydda later during that day.

Evaluation of the situation led to the realization that the Turks would be able to establish a new defence line in the coastal plain only beyond the Auja River. In the Judean hills, the enemy was consolidated in defence of Jerusalem. The situation of the Turkish forces in the hills was not at all an easy one: after the fall of the Junction Station and Jaffa, the only route which could serve the logistic needs of the troops in the Jerusalem area was the Nablus–Jerusalem road. On the other hand, there was only one good road leading to Jerusalem from the coastal plain, thus enabling the Turkish forces to check any future advance of EEF units towards Jerusalem. The conclusion reached from the evaluation of the situation was that the enemy should be attacked immediately and not be allowed to reorganize and establish itself along new lines of defence.

The C-in-C also had to consider the issue of supplies for his advancing forces. Though the capture of Jaffa provided a good way of supplying the forces with the help of the Royal Navy, and the taking of the Junction Station enabled the formation of a railhead there, this would still not solve the logistic problems of the advancing forces. During future operations in the Judean hills, supplies from the railhead would be delivered to the troops by camel convoys.

On 17 November the XXI Corps began its advance into the Judean hills, led by the mounted divisions. The Yeomanry Division left Ramle and made its way to Beit Ur et Tahta. The immobile section of the 8th Mounted Brigade Field Ambulance was located at Annabe, while the 6th Mounted Brigade Field Ambulance immobile section was left in reserve for the advance. According to the plan, casualties from the field ambulance were to be evacuated to Ramle by sand carts. However, it was soon obvious that during operations in the hills the sand carts were useless and casualties could be evacuated almost solely by *cacolet* camels. All available camels were given to the three bearer sections of the division.

The main activities on 18 November took place in the coastal area, where the ANZAC Division captured Sarona, Mulebbis, and Wilhelma without any opposition. ANZAC patrols crossed the Auja River at Hadra on the 19th, reaching Rantie. That was also the day on which the infantry divisions of the XXI Corps began their advance towards the Judean Hills. Latroun and Emmaus were captured by the 232nd Brigade of the 75th Division during the morning, while the 8th Mounted Brigade took Beit Ur et Tahta. Neither the 52nd Division nor the 75th Division could bring its artillery up to the front due to the roadless terrain.

The 75th Division's MDS, which had been established at Junction Station after its capture, now served as a relay station for the casualties of the XXI Corps' divisions during their evacuation to the casualty clearing stations about thirty miles away. However, after the capture of Latroun, the route for evacuation by motor ambulance cars was now the Jaffa–Jerusalem road–Latroun–Junction Station, instead of the Jaffa–Deir Sineid road. The 52nd Division located dressing stations along its route of advance at Lydda, Kubab, and Emmaus. The 19th of November also marked the beginning of winter with heavy rains and temperatures that began dropping considerably.

On 20 November the 75th Division faced determined Turkish resistance at Saris which was captured in the afternoon. The next objective was Qaryet el Inab, the village to which the Turkish force from Saris had retreated. Under the cover of a thick fog, the 232nd and the 233rd Brigades of the 75th Division approached the Turkish troops and annihilated them with bayonets. By 1800 Qaryet el Inab, a key post on the way to Jerusalem, was in British hands. That day, the advance of the Yeomanry Division was

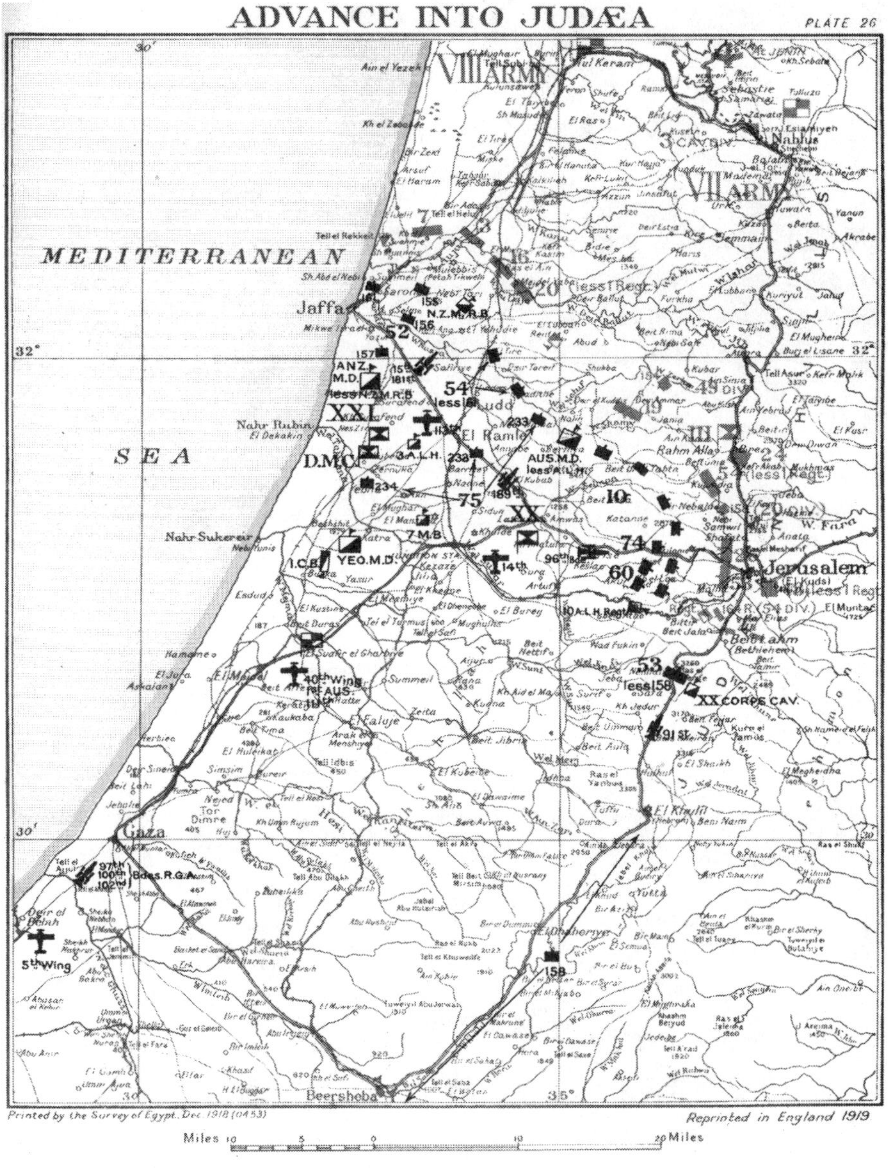

Situation at 6 p.m. on 7-12-17 as known at G.H.Q.E.E.F.

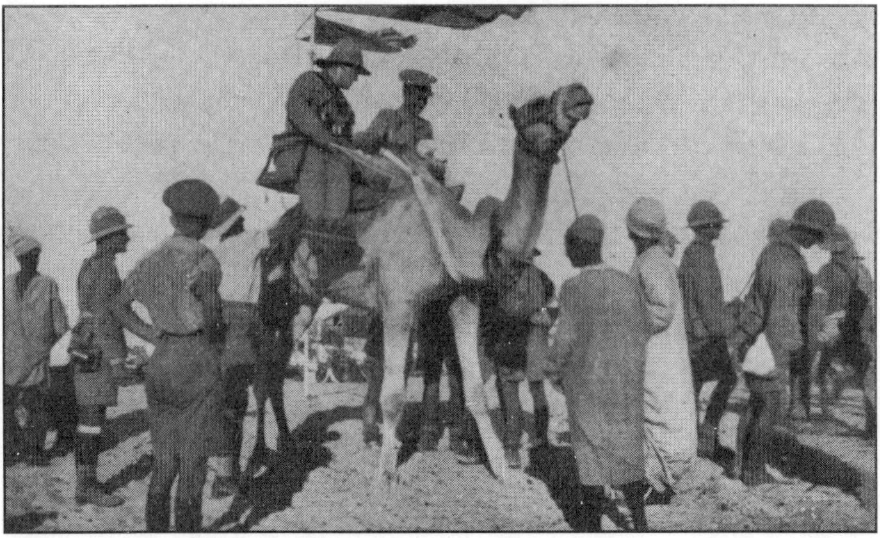

The medical officer going his rounds

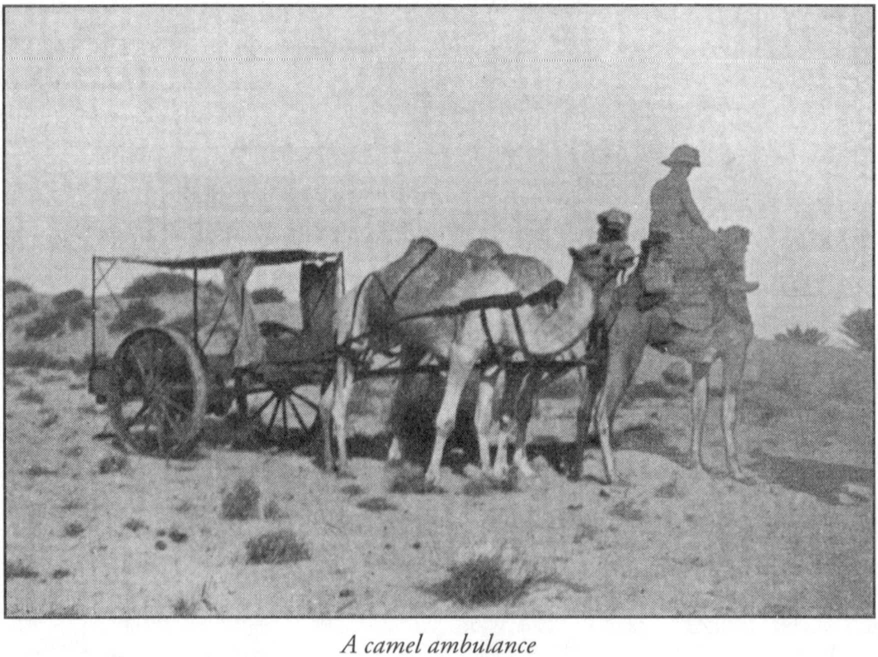

A camel ambulance

checked at Beitunye, about four miles from the Jerusalem–Nablus road, which was the division's objective. It seemed that Turkish resistance was increasing significantly.

The engagements in the Judean hills were entirely different from all previous encounters with the enemy. EEF units fought in mountainous terrain, under very difficult weather conditions, and against strong resistance. The main difference, however, was the issue of medical evacuation. No ambulance transport could travel beyond Annabe, about three miles east of Ramle. Thus, no motor ambulance could approach the collecting stations. Casualties were dressed in regimental aid posts located among rocks or behind boulders, from where they were carried by stretcher-bearers down to valleys or ravines to which *cacolet* camels could be brought. From thence on, the casualties travelled by *cacolet* to Annabe and further on by sand carts to Ramle. Such a trip – from the time of wounding until arrival at Ramle – could last about two days.

At this stage of the campaign many soldiers were sick 'owing to exposure to the cold and inclement weather.'[13] For the first time in the Palestine campaigns several medical officers observed soldiers who suffered from Trench Foot.[14] This was a medical condition caused by exposure to humidity and cold environment while the level of personal hygiene was low, and was common among soldiers engaged in trench warfare in Europe. The condition had not been anticipated as the weather in Palestine was considered to be moderate or even hot. No one had given serious thought to the fact that the winter in the Judean hills was quite cold and might even be freezing.

Between 17 and 23 November the XXI Corps suffered heavy casualties; during 17 November alone the 52nd Division sustained 138 battle casualties from gunshot wounds and 234 casualties due to artillery shells. One of the explanations for this proportion was provided later by an artillery commander who thought that it was typical of a night attack: at night it took the British artillery about 20–30 minutes to counter the Turkish artillery, which in the meantime inflicted many casualties on the attacking infantry battalions.[15] During two unsuccessful attacks on El Jib, the XXI Corps suffered 1,110 casualties: 145 killed, 920 wounded, and 45 missing.

On 20 November the Australian Mounted Division MDS from Julis arrived at Latroun, to be replaced at Julis by the Main Dressing Station of the Yeomanry Division which had arrived from Beit Hanun. On that day, by order of the DMS EEF, No. 75 CCS from Deir el Belah arrived at

Junction Station. Two days later, an improvised train evacuated 200 sitting and 24 lying patients from Junction Station to No. 77 CCS, which had been previously established at Gaza. However, weather conditions became more and more difficult and rain upset everything. Road bridges were destroyed and railroads were washed out. Medical evacuation became an urgent problem, as hundreds of wounded and sick soldiers were congesting the various medical units, mainly the CCS at Junction Station. No. 30 Field Ambulance of the 10th Division, which was at Gaza as a reserve unit, was ordered by the DMS EEF to advance to Junction Station and join the CCS there. When it arrived, it helped a lot by increasing the CCS's capabilities to a great extent. The ADMS of the L-of-C wrote in his diary at that time:

> It did start to rain early in November, but the tracks were fairly firm for the first two weeks, and motor-ambulances could run. As the troops advanced, pushing the Turks before them, our medical arrangements were that the Immobile Sections of the Field Ambulances should stop at convenient sites, whilst the Mobile Sections went on with the advancing troops, sending back their casualties to the Immobile Sections. Then, as railhead advanced, we, of the L. of C. pushed forward a CCS to take over from the Immobile Sections; and they moved again to another site behind the advancing army, remaining there, collecting sick and wounded, until we and the railway overtook them once more. In this way we kept pushing the L. of C. onwards to take over from the G.H.Q. There was thus officially a Casualty Clearing Station at railhead ready always to receive the sick and wounded, and send them back by ambulance train to the nearest stationary Hospital, or even at times to the Base. My administration, therefore, began theoretically with the Casualty Clearing Stations; but I liked to keep in touch with the Immobile Sections of the field Ambulances.[16] [...]
>
> But a worse enemy than the raiding was the rain. It kept pouring night and day. Men who had been sweltering in the heat were now marching north through quagmires, soaking wet, shivering in the thin khaki uniform and shorts they had been wearing in the Sinai Desert.

> The temporary bridges over the Wadi El Arish and the Wadi Guzze had again been swept away by raging torrents. The railway lines sagged. The so-called roads became impassable to wheeled traffic. Evacuation by ambulance became impossible.
>
> The troops, however, were now well through Philistia and across the Jaffa-Jerusalem road. They could send their sick and wounded back to us at 'Junction Station' easily; but, as I have said, we could not evacuate them. They piled up on us. Soon we began to run short of rations, and we had to ask the Field Ambulances to hold their casualties. At length we were compelled to open the emergency stores, and eventually we were down to thirty-six hours' supplies. Our plight, of course, was known. Five hundred camels were assembled hastily at Gaza, and the 30th Field Ambulance battled through the rain and mud to us by forced marches just as our food ran out. Some hundred camels died on the road, but the rest got through. And were we glad to see them!
>
> Luckily there is a short interval between the 'former' and the 'latter' rains, and in this interval we got the sick and wounded back over the reconstructed railway.[17]

The 75th Division advanced on 21 November. The 232nd Brigade captured Qastal and the 234th Brigade took Soba, after resistance. Just before midnight, the 234th also captured the important ridge of Nebi Samweil. But the main forces of the 52nd Division were checked by resisting enemy forces at Beit Ur el Foqa and Beitunye. Several guns were brought forward from Beit Liqiya to Qubeibe to assist the infantry.

The conditions under which the various medical units functioned during that advance were later described in the report of the ADMS 75th Division:

> Up to 1500 hours on 20th, slow progress made up the long 4 mile pass where the advanced dressing stations of 146th Field Ambulance, under desultory shell fire, opened temporary advanced dressing stations along the road at various points. The whole Division, and the transport

> pushing on in heavy mist and rain up the narrow winding route greatly impeded the evacuation of the wounded from the two forward brigades. Darkness came on early and did not improve matters. Orders were issued to 147th Field Ambulance and A Section 123rd I.F.A. to remain at Bab el Wad and the 146th Field Ambulance to push on if it could behind the 232nd and 233rd Brigades who were reported to have entered Qaryet el Inab – the objective – at the point of the bayonets.
>
> 146th Field Ambulance being congested with casualties received from its advanced dressing stations and direct from Units was unable to get beyond Saris, so the only medical unit to enter Qaryet el Inab with the front line Brigades was an advanced dressing station of 147th Field Ambulance under Lieut. Sparrow. Dawn broke on November 21st to disclose both the nakedness of the land, and the exposed position of troops and masses of transport. Owing to the congestion of the latter all along the road from Bab el Wad to Qaryet el Inab, little progress had been made during the night and no Field Ambulances had been able to move up.
>
> Consequently the shelling that took place during the early morning (which caused some 100 casualties to the troops and killed 120 animals in and about the road) caused further delay in the arrival of the field medical units.[18]

During 22 November the British forces repulsed three counter-attacks launched by the Turks at Nebi Samweil. The cost to the four battalions which succeeded in keeping hold of the important post of Nebi Samweil that day was 567 casualties. A British attempt to capture El Jib was repulsed by the enemy. The 8th and the 22nd Yeomanry Brigades had to be withdrawn to Beit Ur et Tahta due to lack of water and supplies.

Next day the 75th Division, supported by artillery, failed to capture El Jib and sustained 480 casualties, including 49 dead. The 5th Mounted Brigade of the Australian Mounted Division reached Ain Karim without real opposition. A third attempt to capture El Jib, this time by the 52nd Division, failed on 24 November. The division suffered 630 casualties during this attack, including

96 dead. On that day the advance of all EEF units in the Judean Hills front came to a halt.

During the last operations of the 75th and 52nd Divisions in the hills northwest of Jerusalem, advanced dressing stations were established at Biddu and Qubeibe, while the main dressing stations for both divisions was located at the monastery of Qaryet el Inab. Medical evacuation from the ADSs was very tedious; whereas the less serious cases were evacuated by *cacolet* camels or on mule-back, the seriously injured had in many cases to be carried by stretcher-bearers to the MDS. Casualties were further evacuated from the MDS by divisional cars to No. 75 CCS at Junction Station. Though the distance between the two medical echelons was only about fifteen miles, the road was so bad and steep that many cars broke down during every journey. By the end of 23 November, only 32 of 53 motor ambulances were available for medical evacuation from Qaryet el Inab.

Throughout that day about 600 cases were treated at the MDS at Qaryet el Inab, but only half of them were able to be further evacuated. During 24 November there were also still 300 casualties waiting for evacuation at the ADS at Qubeibe, the medical evaluation being that about 200 of them were seriously injured. They could not be evacuated since the MDS at Qaryet el Inab was fully occupied and also because of the expected tedious trip which some of them might not survive. For several days the most serious cases stayed at the ADS located at the monastery of Qubeibe, where a surgeon, who had been sent there from the MDS, tended them. There was a shortage of dressings and what was at hand was used for the severe cases. Many soldiers who began, after a long time, to suffer again from septic sores, had to continue to function while their infected lesions were not dressed.[19]

The problem of adequate medical treatment was solved by the RAMC units of the 60th Division. Two of its field ambulances (the 2/5 and 2/6) augmented the ADS at Qubeibe, while a third field ambulance (the 2/4) reinforced the MDS at Qaryet el Inab.[20] In order to solve the urgent problem of evacuation from the dressing stations, 51 sand carts were obtained from the 60th and 10th Divisions, 12 cars were obtained from the 60th Division and 10 more from various sources of the XXI Corps itself. By 27 November the MDS at Qaryet el Inab was cleared and only the most serious cases were still being treated by the surgeon at Qubeibe.

One of the soldiers recorded the misery of being severely wounded at that time:

> What a piteously desolate place the clearing station is! A few tents to house the more desperately wounded lying on the bare earth; whilst those with lesser injuries are scattered about outside, protected against the elements as best these harried medicals are able. Our train of wounded are not welcome, for the staff are overtaxed and unable to give proper attention to those already here. With many grumblings they set to work doing what they can, their grumblings meaningless nothings, for the wounded are far in excess of their facilities and the staff are near exhaustion and the end of their resources. We help to remove the wounded from the camels, then before going in search of stray horses, wander through the tents seeking anyone we may know. In a corner huddled together I found both Miles and Banks, and feel much happier at seeing these two again. Smith followed me in and rolled a cigarette for each with a page from the inevitable Bible. They are not up to talking, but seem to relish a smoke. We tell what news we have, then quietly move out, dodging amongst the many forms lying on the floor. [...]
>
> At the doorway a major grasped my arm. 'I want someone to help me,' he said, 'you look a hefty fellow – come in here, you too,' nodding to Smith.
>
> Lying on a crude board bench was an infantry captain in his shirt only. The trousers had been removed, revealing a shattered leg. When we had looked him over the medical major drew us aside and explained that the leg had to be trimmed, there was no anaesthetic left so it was up to us to hold him down with the aid of the only orderly he could secure.
>
> Smith looked at me then turned to the doctor, telling him that it savoured a little of cruelty. Couldn't some other way be found, or someone else to do it? Apparently there was no other course left, so we decided that if the captain could bear it, we at least could help.

> The doctor explained to the captain what was necessary, that if he was removed in his present condition he would probably not survive it. No objection being raised by the patient, we made the simple preparations required. His good leg we strapped to the slab and threaded a padded rope across his stomach. Smith stationed himself by the leg whilst I placed my arms under his, locking them across his chest, whilst the orderly stood by.
>
> The captain watched our actions with a look of supreme calm till all was ready, then turning his head towards the doctor he quietly told him to get on with it, the first words he had spoken.
>
> With the first cut of the scalpel in the living flesh, the captain gave a shiver and turned his head. I could see into his eyes. They stabbed into me like piercing orbs filled with a depth of agony that I shall not easily forget. I was overcome with an infinite pity for this man, mingled with an admiration for his courage such as few possess [...].[21]

All these medical activities – the treatment of all types of casualties anywhere while giving all units adequate medical support – demonstrate the ability of the EEF medical services to cope with the complex situation imposed by the terrain, the weather, and the battle itself. This ability had been achieved mainly by the proficiency, flexibility, and devotion of the RAMC personnel.

General Allenby realized that in order to resume the advance on Jerusalem, two main issues should be immediately addressed. The first was to relieve the weary divisions of the XXI Corps and replace them with fresh troops. The second was that the time had come to stop pursuing the retreating Turkish Seventh Army into the hills in the direction of Jerusalem. There was a real need for a detailed and thorough plan for the capture of Jerusalem itself. He also addressed the issue of improving communications.

The C-in-C ordered the XX Corps to relieve the XXI Corps in the hills, and the XX Corps units began to reach the arena immediately. On 26 November the 60th Division relieved the 75th Division which withdrew to Latroun, and also the 52nd Division which concentrated at Beit Ur et Tahta. The 2/4 Field Ambulance of the 60th Division arrived at Qaryet el Inab with the 179th Brigade and was set up at the monastery there. The 2/5 and 2/6

Field Ambulances of the 60th Division arrived at Qubeibe with the 180th and 181st Brigades respectively; both were located at the local monastery.[22]

Major H.F. Humphreys, the DADMS of the Yeomanry Division, which suffered relatively less than other units, would write in his diary:

> On the whole the ADMS and I were well satisfied with the way the medical worked, and so apparently was the General. We had always seemed to be living from hand to mouth with a breakdown in sight, but it had never come, and every casualty of the campaign had been promptly evacuated except in the case of captured positions like Beitunia and Zeitoun. The resources at our command had been slender and our casualties extremely heavy in proportion, and when we heard later on of the temporary breakdowns that the other divisions had suffered we began to think we might have fared worse.[23]

During the next days, until the afternoon of 29 November, Turkish forces attacked British units along all sectors of the various fronts. On 25 November they counter-attacked the NZMR Brigade north of the Auja River, causing the force to return to its southern bank. That same day other Turkish forces counter-attacked British units at Nebi Samweil and at Beit Ur el Foqa and were repulsed. Next day they continued to attack in the Nebi Samweil–Beitunye area and also in the Wilhelma–Rantie area. As a result, the British forces evacuated the Zeitun ridge and Beit Ur el Foqa. An attack on Beit Ur et Tahta was repulsed.

On 28 November the XX Corps took over the line from the XXI Corps and established its HQ at Latroun. Corps transport was augmented by 2,000 donkeys which could carry supplies in the hills better than any other animal. The Royal Engineers units began to construct roads between the various units.

The DDMS XX Corps now assumed responsibility for the medical preparations related to the advance on Jerusalem and its capture. According to the plan, the Holy City would be taken by the 60th and 74th Divisions, while the 10th Division would be in reserve. The mobile sections of the field ambulances would follow their brigades as usual. The immobile sections of the field ambulances of the two divisions were to be set up in suitable buildings at Qaryet el Inab, while the combined immobile sections of the

10th Division would be located at Latroun. The plan called for the motor ambulances of the divisions to be pooled at a Corps Ambulance Park and operated under the orders of the DDMS. Every division would retain only six ambulances. No. 35 Motor Ambulance Convoy would be reinforced by motor ambulances from the XXI Corps, altogether sixty-four cars, to evacuate casualties from Qaryet el Inab to Junction Station.

At Junction Station a Main Evacuation Centre would be established, organized along the same principles as had been the Imara Centre during the Third Battle of Gaza. This meant concentration of several medical units, casualty clearing stations and the immobile sections of field ambulances, to allow for more efficient work and flexibility in organization. Casualties would be evacuated from Junction Station by train, motor ambulance cars, and empty returning supply lorries. It was estimated that about 1,000 casualties, sick and wounded, could be evacuated daily from the centre at Junction Station by trains and ambulances, while 600 more would be evacuated by the returning lorries.[24]

At a corps conference at Yalu, General Chetwode, OC XX Corps, presented his plan for the attack on Jerusalem. He assumed that the previous direction of attack – from the north and northwest – had failed due to lack of roads, transport, and water. According to the new plan, the 60th and 74th Divisions would attack Jerusalem from the west and southwest, coordinated with an attack by the 53rd Division from the south. Specific orders were issued that during the taking of the Holy City no artillery should be used.

The official medical history of the campaign noted the following:

> Between the 13th November and 1st December, 3347 sick and 1974 wounded had passed through the Immobile Sections of the 54th division FA's at Beit Hanun, which was receiving casualties from all divisions of the Corps. The percentage of slightly wounded was exceedingly high, as had been the case also in the fighting around Gaza in the early days of the month. In the period 13th to 20th November only 16% and between 21st November and the 1st December only 11% of the wounds were severe. About 320 wounded and 130 sick of the enemy were also evacuated to Beit Hanun during this period.[25]

During the next days the XX Corps divisions were busy making preparations for the assault on Jerusalem while at the same time they, as well as the XXI Corps divisions, were continuously repulsing local Turkish attacks against various sectors.

The C-in-C visited the units in the field, being aware of the extreme weather conditions under which they were fighting. It was typical of General Allenby that he wrote in a letter to his wife: 'It must be very cold and wet where my advanced troops are fighting; up in the mountains, N.W. and N. of Jerusalem. They find the country very difficult; but they are making progress, though news comes very slowly. Tomorrow I shift my HQ forward, some thirty miles, and I shall live in a tent.'[26]

On 3 December the 229th Brigade of the 74th Division recaptured Beit Ur el Foqa only to withdraw later due to tactical considerations. General Chetwode would recall many years later his encounter with General Allenby on that particular day: 'I was afraid we should not finish the thing by night. He asked me why I did not do what Joshua did. He knew, which I did not, that we were in a place called Upper Beth Horon, it was the exact spot where Joshua said "stand still thou - -." He always had his Bible history by heart.'[27]

On 5 December the 'Mott detachment,' which included the 53rd Division and XX Corps cavalry, began its ascent from the Beersheba area via Hebron to participate in the final attack on Jerusalem. By 7 December the 60th and 74th Divisions were ready for the assault. The 60th Division took the high ground south of Ain Karim near Jerusalem. On that day the XXI Corps assumed responsibility for the coastal sector from Lydda and Ramle in the east to the sea shore at the mouth of the Auja River in the west.

During the final assault against Jerusalem the ADMS GHQ, Major Bagshaw, was at the medical complex located at Junction Station according to plan, controlling the evacuation of casualties from both corps.[28]

On 8 December, under heavy rain and fog, the 74th and 60th Divisions attacked the whole length of the Turkish front from Ain Karim to Nebi Samweil. By 0700 the two divisions reached their first objectives, the villages of Ain Karim, Deir Yasin, and Beit Iksa, and the redoubts covering the Jaffa–Jerusalem road in the area. Despite this promising start, General Chetwode had to halt operations and postpone them to the next day due to the fact that the 53rd Division from the south had not reached the Bethlehem area on time. As a result the right flank of the 60th Division was exposed to the enemy. It was also a wise decision, since the infantry troops were almost exhausted due to the rough terrain and weather conditions. They were advancing under heavy rain and in very cold weather without greatcoats and had to rely on their iron rations and personal water bottles till the next morning.[29] With hindsight, one may say that this was perhaps one of the most important decisions taken during the battle of Jerusalem. It allowed the Turks to evaluate the situation and withdraw from the city during the night. The Turkish retreat most probably saved many lives on both sides. It also prevented the Holy City from being damaged had it become the immediate zone of operations.

During the night of 8 December the Turkish forces withdrew from Bethlehem and Jerusalem. Next day, the Mayor of Jerusalem surrendered the city to Major General John S.M. Shea, OC the 60 Division and British troops entered the city. On 11 December General Allenby formally entered the Holy City.

During the days following the Turkish retreat from Jerusalem and the surrender of the city, the British troops faced only sporadic encounters with the enemy. It seems that most Turkish army units in the area were in very bad shape. The troops lacked supplies, many of the soldiers were sick, they were under continuous British pressure, and their morale was low. A letter found on the body of a dead Turkish Officer might describe the military situation from the perspective of the Turkish troops: 'God has so far granted me health and strength and brought me through, but where can it all end? We are tormented by the English; no rest do we receive, and very little food, and our men are dying in hundreds of disease.'[30]

The British nation rejoiced in the victory at Jerusalem. Some saw it as a 'Christmas present' of which the British were indeed in need. Others tried to compare Allenby's campaign in Palestine and the taking of Jerusalem to a successful crusade, ignoring the basic fact that this campaign was not a religious war fought by Christians against Muslims but by a multinational force, including Muslims, fighting against Ottoman rule. The title 'crusade' was especially despised by General Allenby himself.[31]

The capture of Jerusalem created many new problems for the medical services. Though several hospitals were functioning in the city at that time, their situation was quite bad. All had run out of supplies, many of the staff members had vanished, and those remaining suffered from hunger.[32] Some experts in the fields of epidemiology and tropical diseases were already aware that Jerusalem was an unhealthy city.[33] Its inhabitants were known to suffer from various diseases, mainly gastrointestinal infections. Ailments such as dysentery and typhoid were quite prevalent, but cholera outbreaks had also been recorded in the Holy City in the recent past. During the Great War, Jerusalem experienced an outbreak of typhus with a high mortality rate.[34] Another prevalent epidemic disease was trachoma, a very contagious eye disease.

However, 'the greatest scourge of Jerusalem was malaria.'[35] It was very prevalent, with about 27.3 percent of schoolchildren found to have malaria parasites in their blood during the winter.[36] The problem with malaria was that its prevalent type in Jerusalem and the area was the subtertian – a malignant type, caused by plasmodium falciparum – a lethal disease, mainly for children. The vector of malaria in waterless Jerusalem was anopheles bifurcates, a specific mosquito which adapted its life cycle to cisterns, and in Jerusalem there were many cisterns containing rain water.[37]

In December 1917 Jerusalem, the Holy City, was a very dirty place. Its multi-ethnic community lacked basic knowledge of the principles of health and hygiene and was quite indifferent to this problem. The Ottoman rulers had contributed their share to the situation by neglecting health issues. During the spring of 1916 thousands had died of typhus in southern Palestine, many of them in Jerusalem.[38] Sporadic cases of typhus were diagnosed at Jerusalem all the time; cases were diagnosed at Beitunye, on the way to Jerusalem,[39] and an outbreak of typhus was observed at Jaffa several weeks after it had been taken by the British forces.[40] During the last phase of Ottoman rule in Jerusalem, poverty and misery were so prevalent that prostitution had become a common phenomenon even among the most orthodox sectors of the population. The prevalence of venereal diseases was very high both in Jerusalem and Jaffa.[41] The medical services were facing a great challenge, the eradication of malaria and venereal diseases being only the cardinal issues.[42] When the British entered Jerusalem they faced a starving population in need of urgent support in food and supplies no less than medical treatment and delousing.[43]

Thus, immediately after the occupation of Jerusalem a clean-up campaign was urgently needed. No. 115 Sanitary Section of the XX Corps was assigned the task.[44] The field ambulances of the 60th and 53rd Divisions entered the city and established there advanced and main dressing stations. The combined immobile sections of the ambulances remained in their positions at Qaryet el Inab and Latroun for several more weeks. Several days after the capture of Jerusalem, No. 66 CCS arrived from Deir el Belah and was located at a monastery within the city.

The C-in-C was concerned about the defence of Jerusalem, for the Turkish troops were establishing a new front line several miles north of the city. Although the enemy was not expected to use artillery against the Holy City, the threat of a surprise attack was considered to be serious. To avoid this permanent and eminent threat, an advance northward and eastward of Jerusalem was prepared by General Chetwode. Planned to commence by the end of the month, the offensive was approved by General Allenby.

While the XX Corps units were busy preparing for the offensive, its intelligence officers became convinced that the Turks were planning a counter-attack towards Jerusalem for the exact same dates. Studying the information, General Chetwode concluded that the enemy's plans were in accord with his own and decided to allow the Turks to strike first in order to break their forces with a well directed blow. The enemy attacked as expected on 27 December, its forces were repulsed, and the offensive was a complete failure. The British troops counter-attacked the retreating Turkish forces, eventually reaching the area of Beitin about twelve miles north of Jerusalem where they established a new front line which was able to secure Jerusalem from future surprise attack.

In the two-week period between the 15th and the 29th of December the EEF suffered 1,890 casualties, 238 of whom were killed. The majority of the casualties, 1,360, were sustained during the Turkish counterattack on Jerusalem. This phase of the campaign coincided with a new period of heavy rain. As several weeks earlier, the problem of medical evacuation became acute as roads and bridges were ruined by the streams. The CCS at Jerusalem became overcrowded so, in order to help in its work, the DMS EEF decided to bring to Jerusalem several nurses from hospitals in Sinai and southern Palestine, a decision that quite amazed the ADMS L-of-C who was responsible for the hospitals as well as for the nurses:

> We had pushed the 66th CCS forward to cope with the wounded. It was located in one of the numerous religious buildings, known to be bug-infested, and it was overcrowded with casualties owing to the weather hold-up. [...] The weather had improved, and on my way back to Gaza one morning I was

> passing a group of men repairing the wire road when I saw four ambulances approaching. 'Look,' one of the men shouted in an incredulous voice. 'Look, women!' It was a bevy of nursing sisters on the way up to the 66th CCS. [...] Not only were they white women but they were ministering angels going forward to hardship and possibly danger, to look after their comrades. It was an immense thrill.[45]

The arrival of the nurses in Jerusalem was not only a great professional help to the overstrained medical units in the Holy City. It also created, to some extent, a feeling of 'back to normal life' among the civilian population, as well as the troops.

General Allenby had then to establish a reliable defence line in order to protect Jaffa, which was at the time the main harbour of Palestine and could be used by the Royal Navy for landing supplies in large quantities. Its significance grew with the capture of Jerusalem, which could then be supplied through Jaffa harbour. However, the enemy was establishing a front line, based on the natural barrier of the Auja River, only several miles from the harbour which was in the range of its artillery. As long as the artillery threat existed, the navy did not fully cooperate at Jaffa harbour, preferring to continue landing supplies at the mouth of Nahr Suqreir. It seemed imperative to push the Turks several miles further from Jaffa. During the night of 20 December troops of the 52nd Division, supported by Royal Navy gunfire and the RFC, crossed the Auja River, pushed the Turkish units to the north and east, and established a new line about five miles north of the river. Jaffa was now beyond the range of the Turkish artillery.

The new front line established in late December remained essentially unchanged until the final offensive in September 1918. Both opponents needed time to recuperate, consolidate their troops, and make plans for the future.

In his official despatch after the capture of Jerusalem General Allenby wrote:

> The medical services had also performed admirable work under heavy strain, above all the Field Ambulances of the divisions. Until the capture of Jerusalem the nearest CCS was at Junction Station – and for Mott's detachment at Kharm, reached via Beer

> Sheba – but the difficulties were eased when it was possible to install one in the city itself, so that the wounded could have a comfortable break in their journey down the line.[46]

This dispatch was a natural source of pride for the entire medical service. The various EEF medical units, from the regimental aid stations to the casualty clearing stations and hospitals, had from 31 October until the end of December 1917 treated and evacuated 20,918 casualties, injured and sick, and had done this in the best possible manner under the circumstances. A veritable Herculean task. There were, though, other sources of pride as well: 'It is interesting to record that the first Union Jack to be flown in Jerusalem was hoisted by the 2/6th Field Ambulance, which was the first medical unit to open a dressing station in the Holy City.'[47]

6

RAIDS ACROSS THE JORDAN

'What the wounded men in the cacolets must have suffered during this terrible journey can scarcely be imagined.'

Richard M.P. Preston, *The Desert Mounted Corps* (London: Constable and Co., 1921), 173.

'The men showed great gallantry in rescuing under fire wounded comrades who would otherwise have fallen into the hands of the enemy, carrying them in waterproof sheets up stony hills and across steep and rugged defiles.'

Cyril Falls., *Military Operations Egypt & Palestine, from June 1917 to the End of the War*, vol. 1 (London: HMSO, 1930), 377.

General Allenby's first campaign in Palestine, known as the 'Third Battle of Gaza,' was actually accomplished when Jerusalem fell to the EEF in December 1917. For three more months the British defence lines were defined and established, a process completed on 21 February 1918 when an ANZAC Mounted force took Jericho without battle. Thus, the right flank of the British force was secured for the time. EEF units continued to push northwards to attain control over the Jericho plains. Such control improved the strategic and tactical situation of the EEF to a large extent, as it enabled the establishment of a defence line based on natural obstacles. EEF units also controlled most of the routes leading to the Jordan Valley from the east.

A regional HQ was never established at Jericho itself, most probably due to information concerning health conditions there. The reason might be found in General Allenby's letter to General Robertson, the CIGS: 'We have pushed down into the Jordan valley, and taken Jericho, during the past week. Jericho is a typhus-haunted spot; and I don't occupy the village, but hold the heights above it.'[1]

It was then that Colonel A.E.C. Keble, who had served as DMS EEF since the arrival of General Allenby, was transferred to GHQ in Cairo and a new Surgeon General, William T. Swan, arrived from Europe and was appointed the new DMS EEF. Surgeon General Swan came with vast military medical experience acquired during years at the Western Front. His last assignment had been DDMS VII Corps of the 3rd Army in France, where he had served under General Allenby.[2]

For about nine months, until the beginning of the final campaign, the Palestine front remained quiet except for local and limited military actions. The only exceptions were the two raids across the Jordan during the spring of 1918. The debate concerning the reasons and justification for these raids and their strategic and military results began at the time they were carried out and continues to this very day. There were those who thought that the raids represented a 'far sighted strategy of "mystify, mislead and surprise" ' and 'a part of a plan of deception for the next stage.'[3] T.E. Lawrence believed they had achieved their strategic objectives.[4] Others thought the raids had been a mistake.[5] One of these was Lt-General Sir P. Chetwode, commander of the XXth Corps, who commanded the first raid. Years later he would write: 'These two expeditions of Allenby's across the Jordan were the stupidest thing he did, I always thought, and very risky.'[6]

While campaigning in Palestine, the EEF had not encountered any Arab force. The raid into Transjordan would be the first actual encounter, leading to cooperation between the EEF and the Arab forces participating in the Arab Revolt that were operating southeast of the Dead Sea.

Cooperation began during the early stages of the Great War. British interests in the Middle East led Lord Kitchener to offer Hussein Ibn Ali, the Sherif of Mecca and a respected leader in the Arab world, a conditional guaranty of independence for the Arabs if they would support Britain in its war against Turkey. Negotiations continued between Sherif Hussein and Sir Henry McMahon who promised to support Arab independence if the Hashemite tribe led by Hussein would rise up against the Ottomans. On 14

July 1915 Hussein submitted to the British his terms for opening a campaign against the Turkish army. He demanded from them formal recognition of the independence of the Arabs south of 37 North Latitude. After several weeks of negotiations Britain accepted these terms while Sherif Hussein agreed to the several territorial changes demanded by the British.

In the meantime Great Britain and France were secretly negotiating the future of the Middle East in the post-war period. Both governments shared the assumption that the Ottoman Empire was doomed and might cease to exist at war's end. Both were anxious to secure their interests in the new Middle East. On the 15th and 16th of May 1916 the representatives of Britain and France, Sir Mark Sykes and Georges Picot, reached and signed an agreement that came to be known as the Sykes–Picot agreement. It defined the Arab independent area that would become an Arab state or a federation of Arab states. It also defined the British and the French administrative zones in the Middle East, and Italy too was to receive several concessions in former Ottoman provinces.[7]

Sherif Hussein's goal in his revolt against Turkey was to gain independence from the Ottoman Empire and create a single unified Arab state from Aleppo in Syria in the north to Aden in Yemen in the south. Like others at the time, Hussein was unaware of various other British agreements and promises, including the Sykes–Picot agreement, contracted with or made to various national leaders and ethnic groups that were not compatible with each other.[8]

The Arab Revolt began on 5 June 1916 when the Arabs attacked the Turkish garrison at Medina. Two days later Sherif Hussein proclaimed the independence of the Hejaz. On 10 June 1916 the Ottoman garrison at Mecca surrendered to the rebels and by the end of October Hussein proclaimed himself King of the Arabs. From the end of 1916 the British supported the Arab Revolt with gold, weapons, munitions, and supplies. On 15 December 1916 Great Britain recognized Hussein as King of the Hejaz.

British military intelligence watched the Arab Revolt with much interest, as the power that rose up against the Ottoman Empire might serve the interests of the British Empire in the Middle East. British HQ in Egypt sent two British officers to the Hejaz. The first was Lt-Colonel Stuart F. Newcombe, RE, at the head of a British military mission whose task was to evaluate the capabilities of Hussein's rebel force and support him professionally. After leaving the Hejaz, Colonel Newcombe joined the EEF.[9]

The second officer was Thomas E. Lawrence, later to be known as 'Lawrence of Arabia.' At the time, Lawrence was posted with British military intelligence in Cairo. As he knew a lot about the Middle East in general, and Arabs in particular, his superiors believed that he would be the ideal liaison between the Arab rebels and British HQ in Cairo. On 16 October 1916 Lawrence was sent into the Hejaz desert to report on the various aspects of the new political and military power.

Lawrence's major contribution was to induce Arab leaders to coordinate their revolt with British interests. He also managed to convince them not to try to capture the city of Medina. The very existence of a besieged Ottoman garrison in Medina led to Turkish attempts to supply it, and increased the importance of the Hejaz Railway. On 6 July 1917 an Arab irregular force headed by Lawrence took the important harbour of Akaba, on the Red Sea, by a daring attack. The capture of Akaba became a symbol of the Arab Revolt's success: it induced several Arab tribesmen who had hesitated to join the revolt to do so now. It also changed the Turkish attitude towards the Arab rebels, for the Turkish military authorities now realized that the Arabs had become a real threat to the interests of the Ottoman Empire in the area, especially to the important Hejaz Railway. In addition, the taking of Akaba facilitated the supply of the Arab army by the British.[10]

On 16 January 1918 an Arab force commanded by Feisal, Sherif Hussein's son, seized Tafila, about fifteen miles southeast of the Dead Sea. On 26 January a counterattacking Turkish force suffered heavy losses and was forced to retreat.[11] It was obvious that the Turks would try to capture Tafila again, the considered opinion being that this Turkish move would take place in March. This was the political and military background to the first raid across the Jordan.

THE FIRST RAID

As early as January 1918 General Allenby wrote to the CIGS about his plans concerning a future raid:

> Then I want to extend my right, to include Jericho and the North of the Dead Sea. Later, I hope to be able to push across the Jordan, and throw a big raid, past Salt, against the Hedjaz Railway. If I could destroy 10 or 15 miles of rail and some

> bridges; and get [in] touch with the Arabs under Feisal – even temporarily – the effect would be great. [12]

The raid had several objectives. The first was to support Sheikh Feisal's Arab army. The Arab forces were then concentrated around the Dead Sea and Tafila, intending to take the town of Ma'an. The British realized that by raiding the Amman area the EEF would help the Arabs by diverting Turkish forces from the south to the area being raided. A successful operation might for the first time establish coordination between the Arabs and the EEF.[13]

An operation in the east might also divert the enemy's attention from the coastal area where General Allenby was already contemplating the future final campaign. He also had a practical concern: he thought that the summer climate in the malarial Jordan Valley was severe and that the higher, cooler Es Salt–Amman area was better suited for billeting purposes. Amman might serve as a future base for operations towards Syria, as it could provide the British with much flexibility while denying the Turks the ability to manoeuvre that they so needed.

The raiding force consisted of the 60th Division, the ANZAC Mounted Division, the Imperial Camel Brigade, several batteries of artillery, bridging and pontoon units,[14] together with the necessary logistic and medical units. The force was subordinated to the XX Corps and commanded by Major-General Shea, OC 60th Division, and hence named 'Shea's Force.'

The objectives assigned to Gen. Shea were specified in the orders for the raid issued by the XX Corps HQ on 13 March 1918: to cross the Jordan on 19 March, occupy Es Salt with his infantry, push his cavalry, and destroy the Hejaz Railway at Amman. 'The objectives to be selected on the railway will be such that their destruction will make it impossible for the enemy to use the line for a prolonged period.'[15] After destroying the railway, the 'Shea Force' was ordered to leave a garrison, a strong detachment with reliable communications, at Es Salt. The rest of the force was to withdraw west of the Jordan River.

The route chosen for the raid was Ghoraniye–Shunet Nimrin–Es Salt–Amman. This meant a difficult climb of about 4,000 feet along fifteen miles, from the Jordan Valley level to Es Salt, most probably under enemy fire. Supplies were brought by train to Jerusalem and from there to Jericho by lorries which continued to the Jordan crossings, from where every division was responsible for its own logistic arrangements. The divisional transport trains

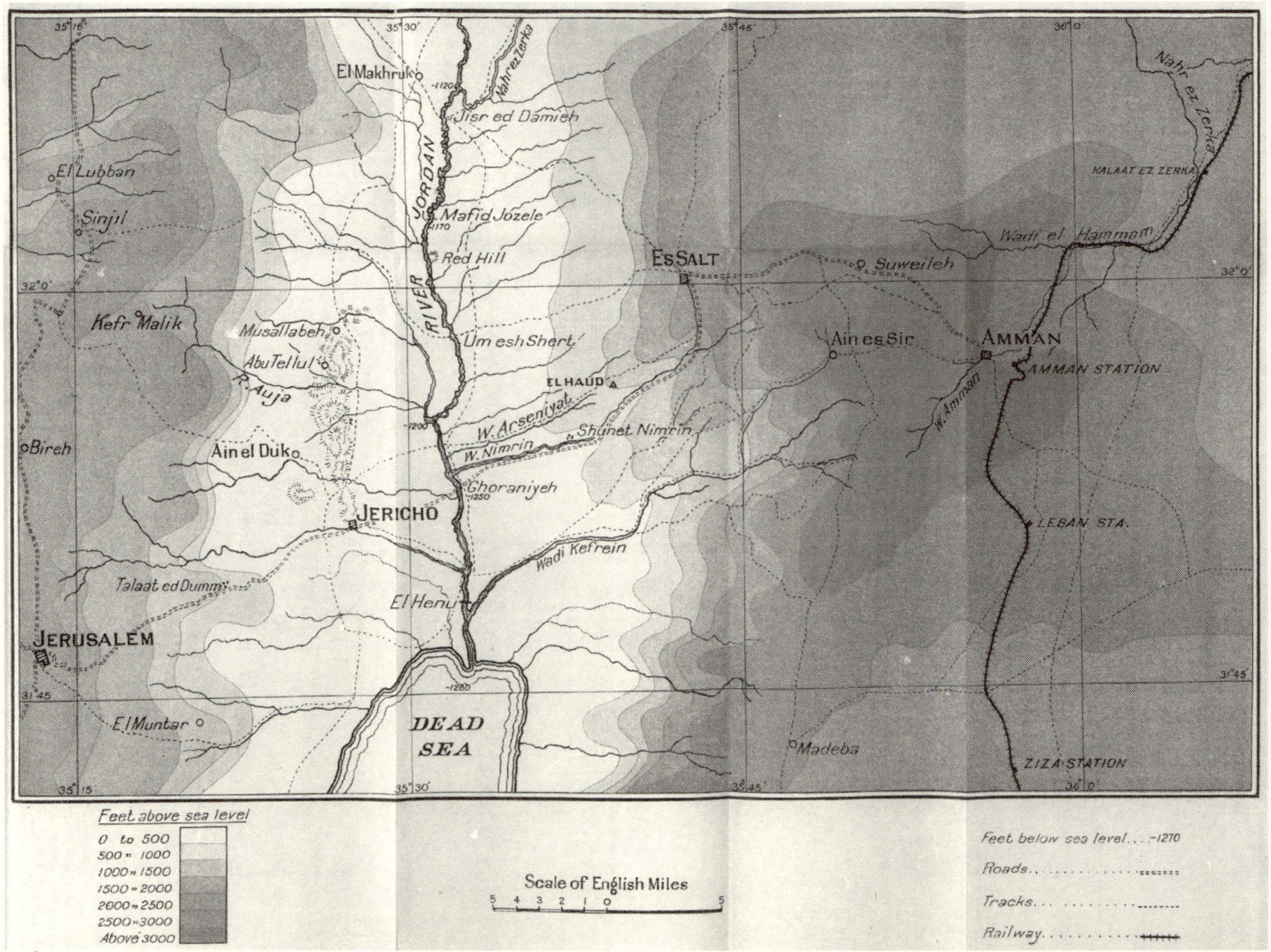
El Makhruk
Jisr ed Damieh
Nahr ez Zerka
JORDAN
RIVER
Mafid Jozele
Red Hill
El Lubban
Sinjil
Es Salt
Suweileh
Kefr Malik
Musallabeh
Abu Tellul
R. Auja
Um esh Shert
El Haud
W. Arseniyat
Shunet Nimrin
W. Nimrin
Ain es Sir
AMMAN
AMMAN STATION
W. Amman
Wadi el Hammam
KALAAT EZ ZERKA
Bireh
Ain el Duk
Ghoraniyeh
JERICHO
Wadi Kefrein
LEBAN STA.
Talaat ed Dumm
El Henu
JERUSALEM
El Muntar
DEAD SEA
Madeba
ZIZA STATION
Feet above sea level
0 to 500
500 " 1000
1000 " 1500
1500 " 2000
2000 " 2500
2500 " 3000
Above 3000
Scale of English Miles
Feet below sea level ... -1270
Roads
Tracks
Railway

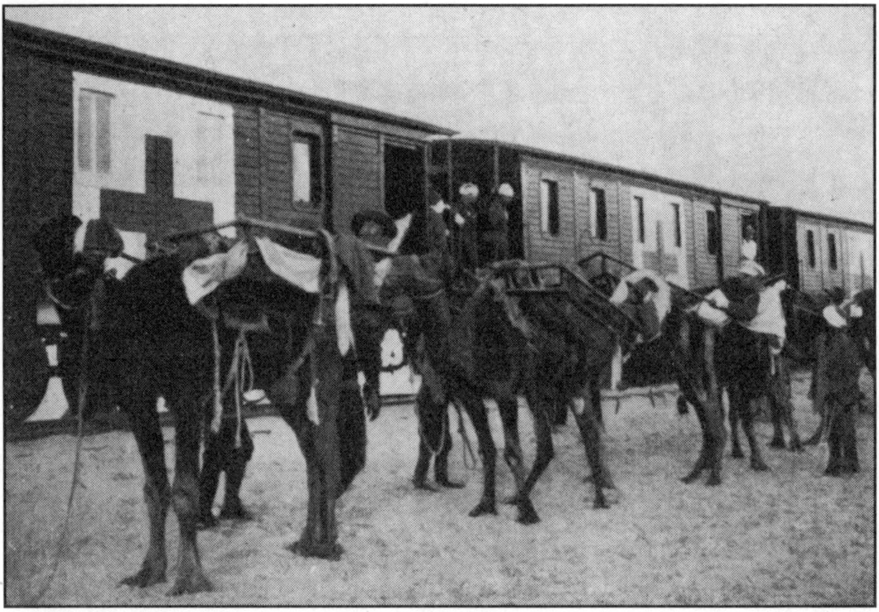

Desert hospital train

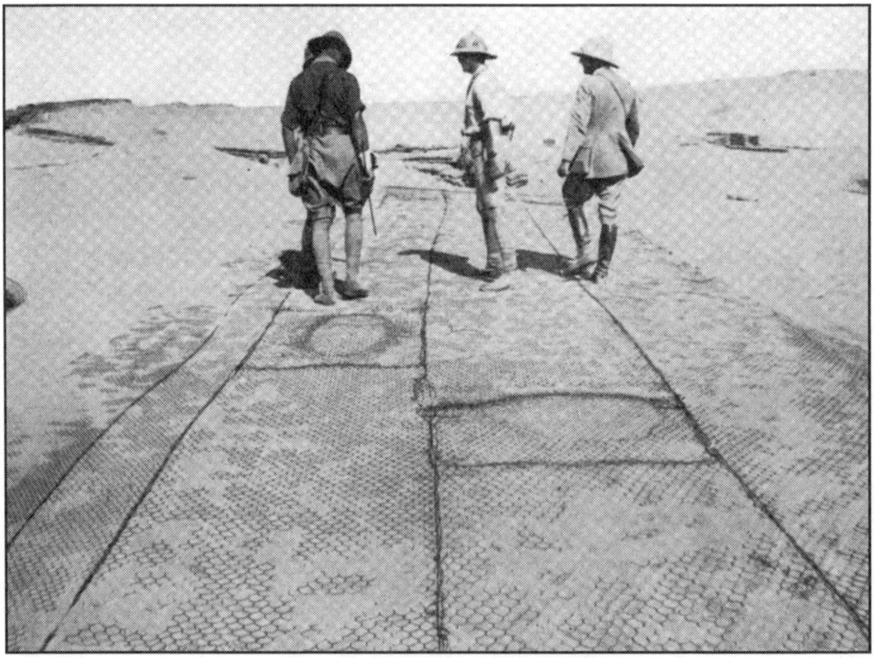

Wire netting track acrosss the Sinai Desert

conveyed supplies along the main road as far as Shunet Nimrin. The ANZAC Division was reinforced by three loaded camel convoys, each consisting of 550 camels. One convoy carried supplies for the first phase of the raid, an attack on the Shunet Nimrin–Es Salt road. The other two carried one day's supplies to the Amman area. The 60th Division was reinforced by two camel convoys, each consisting of 805 camels for Es Salt. The lessons of past operations having been learnt, this time there was plenty of water and enough grazing pasture for the horses and camels.

The medical plan was very comprehensive and attempted to anticipate possible medical problems during various stages of the raid. It also took into account the dimensions of space and time which might influence the evacuation and treatment of sick and wounded soldiers and prisoners of war. For example, the plan assumed that a medical unit might support several combat units fighting in the same area for a certain period of time and not just the units to which it had been assigned.

The brigades were followed by the mobile sections of their field ambulances whose wagons and sand carts were all concentrated near Jericho, under the control of the two participating ADMSs. They were expected to follow the brigades when circumstances would permit. The ADMSs had at their disposal three tent subdivisions and 150 *cacolet* camels, a transport unit which would suffice for the treatment and evacuation of 150 casualties. The 60th Division field ambulances were augmented by the 1/1st Field Ambulance of the 53rd Division under Colonel E.B. Dowsett, ADMS 60th Division.[16]

Medical equipment for the field ambulances was transported by camels since the roads were expected to be impassable for wheeled vehicles. The regimental medical equipment was carried by packhorses. Thirty five *cacolet* camels were allotted to each field ambulance. The personnel of the cavalry field ambulances were all mounted except for that of the tent subdivisions.

The MDS for the whole force, consisting of the tent subdivisions of two field ambulances of the 60th Division under the command of Lt-Colonel T.B. Layton, was located at Jericho. Attached to it were the Desert Mounted Corps Operating Unit and the consulting surgeon to the EEF, Colonel Henry Wade. This crucial medical unit, which had already distinguished itself during the battle for Beersheba, was under the direct command of the DDMS XX Corps, Colonel Richard H. Luce.

The motor ambulances and the horsed ambulance wagons were parked near Jericho under command of the DADMS ANZAC Mounted Division.

The intention was to use them for evacuation of casualties from the ANZAC Mounted Division ADS, planned to be opened during the first stage of the operation, and the main dressing station at Jericho. It was also planned that during the second phase of the battle another MDS would be opened at Shunet Nimrin to receive all cases evacuated from forward medical units. At Tal'at-ed-Dumm, halfway between Jericho and Jerusalem, a medical post was set up by a field ambulance from the 53rd Division as a rest station for the casualties on their way to Jerusalem. Two casualty clearing stations were located in buildings in Jerusalem itself, ready to receive casualties and continue their treatment. Just prior to the raid, both the DMS, Major-General Swan, and the DDMS XX Corps, Colonel Luce, visited the various medical units and found everything in order.[17]

The raid, planned to begin on 19 March, was put off to 21 March due to heavy rains and low temperatures which turned the rain into sleet. Surprise was crucial to the raid's success and the delay, no doubt, was among the factors contributing to the loss of surprise and therefore jeopardized the entire operation. During the night of 21 March the operation began by crossing the Jordan which was flooded. The crossing was very difficult and the progress of the infantry units very slow, as heavy rains continued and the ground was slippery and exceedingly rough. Weather conditions and the difficult terrain made participation of most of the artillery units impossible. Es Salt was taken by the 1st Australian Light Horse Brigade only on the eve of 25 March. Several attempts by the mounted units to take Amman or to cause substantial damage to the Hejaz Railway near that city failed due to enemy resistance.

The medical units of the 60th Division which entered Es Salt encountered some unexpected health problems:

> In Es Salt we found four private houses used as a Turkish hospital, and full of sick and wounded Turks, with one badly wounded British POW of the 53 division. The total in these four houses was ninety, and included twenty four suffering from typhus.
>
> During the short interval between the retreat of the Turks and the entry of the British, the civilian population looted the hospital of everything they could carry off, even to the bedding of the patients.[18]

On 29 March the water level of the Jordan rose, all bridges with the exception of the Ghoraniye bridge were swept away, and there was a real threat to the L-of-C. This was the last in the cascade of events happening to the force while the enemy in the Amman area was being reinforced by fresh troops. The prospects of achieving the raid's objectives were diminishing by the moment.

On 30 March the C-in-C decided to retreat from Amman.[19] The retreat under enemy fire was very arduous: for about ninety hours the troops marched and fought continuously without sleep or rest. There was an extreme shortage of supplies despite the good planning and preparations. The camels could not keep pace with the needs and many of them succumbed to the horrible weather and difficult terrain. Most of the time the troops were without tents or shelter of any kind.

Operation of the Medical Services

The number of casualties suffered during the first raid into Transjordan was 1,348. They were treated at the various medical echelons according to the severity of their injuries and were then evacuated west of the Jordan River. The wounded suffered severely during the process of evacuation, which fortunately worked according to plan. The battle casualties from the firing line near Amman were borne on light stretchers and blankets to the regimental aid posts which were located about half a mile behind the front. From there they were evacuated by sand carts to the ADSs which were established about three miles to the rear of the regimental aid posts. The round trip by sand carts took about three to six hours. The next stage in the voyage of the sick and wounded was evacuation to the ANZAC Divisional Collecting Station which served as an MDS and was located about six miles further back, at Birket Umm Amud. The terrain was so rough that evacuation from the ADS to the Divisional Collecting Station was only possible by *cacolet* or on horseback. As the journey between these two stations lasted about six to seven hours, two more dressing stations were established on the route between them to allow medical examination of the casualties and redressing if necessary. The agony of the wounded did not escape the notice of their peers:

> Every seriously wounded man had therefore to be carried from Amman to Es Salt on the camel cacolets. It would be scarcely

> possible to devise a more acute torture for a man with mutilated limbs than this hideous form of ambulance-transport.[20]
>
> As no satisfactory contrivance had been evolved to make the camel cacolets suitable for patients with fractures of the thigh treated by means of the Thomas Splint, the latter were applied only at the Divisional Collecting Station, where also the treatment of shock caused by the long trip and without fixation of the fractured limb, was treated.[21]

The alternative transportation, on horseback, was not much better:

> Beds of greatcoats, freely offered, were built-up on each horse and the wounded were placed face down with their heads to the horses' tails. Their hands were then tied under the flanks, and their feet secured in nose-bags at the front. In this fashion they were borne for twelve miles.[22]

The road from the Divisional Collecting Station to the west was passable by wheeled transport, and evacuation was continued to the 60th Division Advanced Dressing Station at El Howeij, five miles to the rear of Es Salt. During a later stage of the operation, before the retreat, this station was united with the ANZAC Division Receiving Station located east of Es Salt. The time spent in actual evacuation from the firing line to the Main Dressing Station at Jericho was about twenty-four hours for these forty-five miles. Three more hours were needed for the voyage from Jericho to Jerusalem.

On 31 March there were over 240 casualties at the Divisional Collecting Station, and their evacuation seemed to be a crucial task of all units at that time in order to avoid the risk of abandoning any wounded soldier in enemy territory. Thus, all available means were recruited from both divisions. The collecting station was reinforced and could now begin the retreat with its patients being under medical supervision. Fifty casualties were sent to the rear on foot.

The retreat of all units, especially of the loaded medical units, was very tedious due to the cold weather, heavy rain, and mud. When daylight broke on 1 April, Turkish cavalry drew near the medical convoy and opened fire. At one instance the enemy got between the covering party and the ambulance men. As most of the casualties were loaded on horses they managed to escape, except for two mortally wounded who were left behind and eventually died. The withdrawal was completed by the evening of 2 April.[23]

The XX Corps MDS at Jericho was one of the highlights of the medical plan. An essential part of this unit was the Desert Mounted Corps Operating Unit that had been established after the Second Battle of Gaza. This special unit served as a prototype for several other mobile operating units which had been approved by the DMS, Major-General Swan, for the EEF. It was typical of the cooperation among units and personnel in the EEF that this unit was ordered to Jericho, where it served under the DDMS XX Corps. Located at Jericho and supervised by the EEF surgical consultant, Colonel Henry Wade, the surgeons at the unit had both the experience and the equipment needed to give the best surgical treatment in any urgent case in which it was indicated.

The operating unit at Jericho performed ninety-six operations on urgent cases evacuated from beyond the Jordan. Thirteen of them suffered from abdominal or pelvic injuries, ten from chest injuries, and eleven from head injuries. Another eighteen patients suffered from large flesh wounds and most of the rest from wounds and fractures of limbs. Thirty-six men in this group also suffered multiple injuries. The mortality rate among the cases operated on was ten (10.4 percent). Considering the fact that only urgent cases underwent surgery at the advanced operating unit and that most of them had been injured many hours before reaching the operating theatre, the results were quite impressive.

The medical arrangements and the work done at the Advanced Operating Unit were highly appreciated, even by laymen: 'At Jericho there was an operating unit for serious cases, and there is no doubt that this unit saved the lives of many by an immediate operation, who would almost certainly have died had they been sent straight on to Jerusalem.'[24] During the raid 988 casualties and 1,471 sick soldiers were treated and evacuated by the various medical echelons.[25] Nearly two thousand patients, including sick soldiers and sick and wounded prisoners of war, were evacuated in this way during the operation. The first raid across the Jordan was one of the very few actions in which the cavalry sustained more casualties than did the infantry, about two thirds of the casualties being from the ANZAC Mounted Division.

A letter sent by General Allenby to the War Office, written during April 1918, might throw some light on the relations between British and Turkish-

German units at the front. Such relations were the outcome of generally mutual respect for international codes and conventions.

> The statement that I requested armistice is not correct, but is probably founded on following: -
> On 11th April, Germans with Red Cross flags appeared at 0 98 S 26 C; they collected dead and wounded and were not fired on. Later, 4th Welsh Regiment sent out stretcher bearers to same locality, they were, however, fired on and retired as did Germans.
>
> On 15th April, Officer Commanding 3/3rd Gurkha Rifles sent out a Red Cross flag with two men to look for wounded. A German Officer met them and a dividing line and an hour was fixed for the following day.
>
> On 17th April a Medical Officer and burying party were sent out and an enemy medical officer and burying party also appeared. Proceedings watched by OC 1/4th Bn. Wiltshire Regiment. There was no contact between parties, and except where these parties were at work no cessation of artillery or rifle fire. When burying was finished a German officer came forward under Red Cross flag and handed over pay books and identity discs of certain men of 3/3rd Gurkha Rifles whom he had buried. German officer stated Lieutenant W.F. Patton, 3/3rd Gurkha Rifles, was a prisoner and unhurt, having been stunned by a shell. Our party did not bury any enemy dead.[26]

THE SECOND RAID

Less than four weeks had passed before another incursion into Transjordan was undertaken, but the situation was quite different on the eve of the second raid. On 21 March 1918, the day on which the first operation was commenced, the massive German 'Ludendorff Offensive' began on the Western Front.[27] As a result of the perilous situation at that front General Allenby was ordered to immediately transfer to Europe two of his most experienced infantry divisions and some of his artillery units. He was also ordered to freeze any offensive initiative till the autumn and to concentrate on the defence of

Palestine. Thus, twenty-four experienced British battalions from four infantry divisions (10th, 53rd, 60th, 75th) were sent to France. An additional ten battalions were broken up to reinforce the remaining British battalions. The units that had been sent to Europe were replaced by thirty-three Indian battalions. Twenty of them arrived directly from India, lacking any previous combat experience, while the other thirteen were formed in Palestine. The four infantry divisions were rebuilt on the Indian model: every division now consisted of nine Indian battalions and three British battalions.[28] All this meant that since the beginning of April 1918 the EEF was in the midst of a process of reorganization. This included mainly training the recently arrived Indian units and their incorporation into the already existing divisions and assignments.

The second changed circumstance concerned the military situation in Transjordan. Since 11 April, the Arab forces were engaged in continuous fighting against the Turkish units guarding the Hejaz Railway near the southern town of Ma'an. The Arabs managed to destroy several sections of track and railway stations in that area. As the railway was very important to the Turkish army, it was expected that Turkish forces from the Amman area would be transferred to Ma'an. Not only could such a move put a stop to any further activities of the Arab force, but might also threaten its very existence.

To prevent the Turks from transferring forces from the Amman area, on 18 April Major-General Edward W.C. Chaytor, commander of the ANZAC Division, was ordered to harass their forces along the Jordan. It was assumed that this would induce the enemy to believe that a new attack on Amman was imminent and prevent the despatch of any Turkish reinforcements towards Ma'an. In the meantime the second raid was planned for mid-May.

One of the results of both the first raid and the harassment by the 'Chaytor Force' during April was that the enemy did indeed become convinced that another attack against Amman would soon be mounted. This led to reinforcement and entrenchment of the Turkish forces in Shunet Nimrin, who were then on constant alert. The Turks also repaired and reconstructed the roads leading from Es Salt and Ein es Sir to Shunet Nimrin, being the only route of supply for their force dug in at the front in that area.

The last, but not the least, of General Allenby's considerations was a message from the Bani Sakhr Arab tribe which controlled the area of Madaba to the east of the Dead Sea. According to this message, they were more than willing to participate in a future campaign against the Ottoman forces in Transjordan, if such an action would take place before 4 May. General Allenby had planned to raid the Es Salt region anyway, and communication and cooperation with the Arab forces was one of the objectives of such a future operation. The Bani Sakhr message only hastened the events to come.

The objectives of the second raid were similar to those defined for the first, to which General Allenby added another: 'To seize the first opportunity to cut off and destroy the enemy's force at Shunet Nimrin, and, if successful, to hold Es Salt till the Arabs could advance and relieve my troops.'[29] It was understood that destruction of the Turkish force at Shunet Nimrin and extension of the British lines to the Moabite hills could present an opportunity to spend the summer not in the hot Jordan Valley, but rather in a healthier and more comfortable area.

The force assembled for the second operation was larger than that which had participated in the first raid. It included the Australian and the ANZAC Mounted Divisions, the 60th Infantry Division (minus the 181st Brigade), the Imperial Camel Brigade, an Indian cavalry brigade, an Indian infantry brigade, and several artillery, engineering, and medical units. This time the forces were under the direct command of the Desert Mounted Corps.

According to the plan, the first stage would be a heavy artillery bombardment of the Turkish units occupying areas along the Jordan and Shunet Nimrin. In the next stage, the 60th Division would attack the enemy's entrenched force at Shunet Nimrin, on the main route to Es Salt. If this proved successful, the ANZAC Mounted Division was then scheduled to break through the enemy's right flank and ascend the hills towards Es Salt.

The task of the Australian Mounted Division, reinforced by cavalry brigades from the ANZAC Division, was to cross the Jordan over the Ghoraniye bridge and move rapidly along the eastern bank of the river to reach the Damiye Bridge and secure it. By this act the cavalry force would achieve two goals: the first was to prevent any enemy reinforcements from the western side of the Jordan, the other was to gain control of all routes leading to Es Salt from the Jordan Valley. Then it was to move to Es Salt as soon as possible, around the enemy's right flank, by a rapid advance through the hills. The Imperial Camel Brigade's task was to protect the bridgeheads at Auja and Um Shert.

One result of the decision to cooperate with the Bani Sakhr tribe was that preparation for the operation was done hastily and the time allowed for assembling the participating units was too short, as several of them were training in remote areas.

Since the arena of the second raid was not much different from that of the first one and the objectives were similar, the logistical plan was along the same lines as that prepared for the previous raid. It was extended somewhat, as it had to provide for larger participating forces. The problem of food for the horses, camels, and mules was much facilitated by the fact that at this time of the year there was ample natural pasture for grazing and the brooks in the area were full of drinking water. The main routes were in better condition than before because the rains had ceased and the Turkish army had managed to repair some of the damage caused by the weather. This was also considered an advantage for the enemy, as it increased its potential flexibility in shifting units from one arena to another.

The medical plan for the raid was based on the regimental medical units, the mobile sections of the field ambulances, and on Main Dressing Stations under the responsibility of the Desert Mounted Corps DDMS, Colonel Rupert M. Downes. Though the medical units of the Australian and the ANZAC Mounted Divisions were not short of personnel, they were all under-strength in camels and *cacolets*. This problem was solved by the DMS who ordered reinforcing these medical units with *cacolet* camels from the XX Corps. Due to the short time available for the preparations, these camels arrived too late, many of them only when the raid had already begun and some even after it was over.

The medical plan called for every regimental aid post to be reinforced by bearers from the corresponding field ambulance. As a lesson of the first raid, the mobile sections of the field ambulances were organized to carry as much equipment as possible on packhorses. The field ambulances of the Indian brigades lacked any real combat experience, were under-staffed, and under-equipped. According to the plan, the immobile sections of the 1st and 2nd Australian Light Horse Field Ambulances would only arrive on the scene on the third day of the raid.

The Corps Main Dressing Station at Jericho was also reinforced this time. It now consisted of two tent subdivisions of field ambulances of the 60th Division and one section of the 121st Indian Field Ambulance. Attached to it was the Desert Mounted Corps Operating Unit reinforced by a surgical team from the Citadel Hospital in Cairo and Colonel H. Wade, the surgical consultant of the EEF. To this unit were also attached two 'malarial diagnosis stations' whose task, while receiving sick soldiers suffering from fever, was to diagnose if they suffered from malaria so as to initiate treatment as soon as possible. It was expected that until such cases were admitted to the Corps Main Dressing Station, the personnel of these units could help the other teams treat battle casualties. Three ANZAC dental officers and the personnel of the ANZAC field laboratory were also attached to this unit. From the Corps MDS at Jericho, the sick and wounded soldiers were further evacuated to the casualty clearing stations in Jerusalem.

The second raid into Transjordan began on the night of 29 April with a local tactical surprise: the Australian Mounted Division moved towards the Ghoraniye bridge, leaving all the camp lights on. Simultaneously, units of the 52nd Division from the XX Corps operated along the western bank of the Jordan and captured a local village in an attempt to create a diversion.

The Australian Mounted Division forces began to cross the Jordan at 2200, and at dawn they were already near the Umm Shert bridge on their way to secure the Damiye bridge area. While one Light Horse brigade was ascending from Umm Shert to Es Salt, another one was left at the Damiye area and the rest of the force approached Es Salt from the northwest. By the evening of 30 April, the first day of the raid, the 3rd Australian Light Horse Brigade took Es Salt while two other Australian Light Horse Brigades were making their way to that town.

During the same night, the 60th Division three times unsuccessfully attempted to break through the entrenched enemy lines at Shunet Nimrin, suffering many casualties. No advance was achieved by repeated attacks of the infantry units during 30 April. The outcome of the 60th Division's repeated attempts to destroy the Turkish force at Shunet Nimrin was that the main road from Shunet Nimrin to Es Salt could not be used by the Turks. On the other hand, due to the failure to break through the Turkish line at Shunet Nimrin this road, which had been planned as the main supply route, was never in British hands. This caused some logistic problems as the camel convoys could not bring supplies from the depot near Jericho, through the bridgehead, to some distant units. The main problem was lack of ammunition.

On 1 May a decisive and powerful full scale counter-attack was launched by the enemy, mainly at the Damiye bridge and along the Jordan Valley. Turkish army units were also approaching the Es Salt area. Several British brigades found themselves in very dangerous situations, the worst being that of the 4th Australian Light Horse Brigade. It was attacked on three sides, including by a force which had crossed the Jordan on a new bridge whose existence was unknown to British intelligence. The brigade was pushed to the mountains trying hard to protect at least the route from Es Salt to Umm Shert which now became the only available route of communications and retreat for the cavalry units. The Bani Sakhr tribe fighters, whose role in the operation could now be very helpful, never showed up and did not participate in the campaign.

In trying to avoid unnecessary confrontation with superior enemy forces, several artillery guns were abandoned. 'These were the only guns lost to the enemy during the long campaign in Palestine,'[30] a fact that spoke for itself about the situation. Several wagons, ambulance cars, and supplies were also lost to the enemy. It became obvious that the objectives of the operation could not be achieved. During the afternoon of 3 May, General Allenby ordered the retreat from Es Salt.

Whereas during the first part of the raid cavalry units were ordered to attack the Turkish Force at Shunet Nimrin from behind in order to help the infantry division succeed in its frontal assault, things were changed in its later stages. Then, the severe situation of the Australian Mounted Division dictated an inversed approach: Major-General Shea, commander of the 60th Division, was ordered to attack again in Shunet Nimrin, his objective this time being a diversion to enable the cavalry units to withdraw from Es Salt and from the hills. At the same time, and with the same intention, British airplanes dropped 600 lbs. of bombs on Amman, reporting direct hits on the railway station.

The Australian Light Horse units began to withdraw under fire in difficult terrain. 'The men showed great gallantry in rescuing under fire wounded comrades who would otherwise have fallen into the hands of the enemy, carrying them in waterproof sheets up stony hills and across steep and rugged defiles.'[31] By 0220 AM on 4 May, the evacuation of Es Salt was complete. At 1500 on the same day the last cavalry troops crossed the Jordan at Ghoraniye and by nightfall all three divisions were west of the river, leaving only bridgeheads for future activities.

Operation of the Medical Services

As the forces crossed the Jordan during the night of 29 April, a Divisional Receiving Station was established by the ANZAC Mounted Division at the bridgehead at Ghoraniye. The Australian Mounted Division Receiving Station moved forward with units of the division with the intention of being activated on the Shunet Nimrin–Es Salt road, above Shunet Nimrin, after the latter had been taken. It was planned that casualties from this station would be evacuated to the Main Dressing Station at Jericho, a distance of about six miles, by motor ambulances of the 4th Cavalry Division. A Divisional Collecting Station was located by the Australian Mounted Division two miles east of the Jordan on the Umm Shert–Es Salt track.

The 3rd and 4th Australian Light Horse Field Ambulances followed their brigades, first northward to the Damiye bridge area and then along the road from Damiye to Es Salt. The two medical units came under heavy shelling along this route. While the 4th Australian Light Horse Brigade was fighting in the Damiye area, its field ambulance established an ADS three miles north of Umm Shert to serve both the 3rd and the 4th Australian Light Horse Brigades. The 3rd Australian Light Horse Field Ambulance followed its brigade along the difficult track into the hills towards Es Salt, using only its horses and camels as the track was impassable for any wheeled vehicle. This unit halted for the night in a wadi four miles from Es Salt.

The 1st Australian Light Horse Field Ambulance followed its brigade, without any transport animals. The 2nd Australian Light Horse Field Ambulance moved behind its brigade and managed by evening to get to Es Salt with nine of its *cacolet* camels. The 5th Light Horse Field Ambulance followed its brigade up the Umm Shert–Es Salt track, leaving behind its vehicles and camels, as the route was too steep for them to traverse. By the end of the first day of the operation, when night fell on the five exhausted cavalry brigades and their field ambulances around Es Salt, their medical evacuation ability was very limited: only twenty-nine *cacolet* camels of the 2nd and 3rd Light Horse Field Ambulances. A number of captured German cars and other motor vehicles were given to the medical units for this purpose by the combat units.

At the Shunet Nimrin front three advanced dressing stations handled the casualties before transferring them further to the divisional receiving station. As the distances were short and the battle static, the casualties reached the divisional receiving station three hours after the fighting had begun. Two hours later they were admitted to the Corps Main Dressing Station at Jericho. Those who were not in need of urgent operations there, who naturally were the majority, were transported to the CCSs in Jerusalem by twenty eight heavy and ten Ford motor ambulances which had been ear-marked for this purpose. The round trip took about seven hours.

Until evening of the first day of the raid, 409 casualties were admitted to the ANZAC Mounted Division Receiving Station. Medical evacuation from this station went smoothly and was very efficient, utilizing any available vehicle at the bridgehead. Due to this efficiency the Divisional Receiving Station was clear of patients most of the time, ready to receive future casualties. A medical officer wrote the following in one of his letters:

> We took over the town [Es Salt], our men bivouacked in the big square and our headquarters seized a quite good building the former German soldiers' home. My work began at once. I heard there was a hospital in the place, and on visiting it I found it was the previous Turkish-Boche hospital, and had for one day taken over by a Red Cross officer and then left to a sanitary squad. I thereupon took command and found some forty British West Indian black soldiers of our own, and forty odd wounded Turks and about twelve Australian accident casualties. There were dressings, drugs, splints, or utensils. I did find, however, a signalling apparatus in a cupboard and some rifle grenades in a drawer. The native attendant told me that the signalling apparatus had been in constant use from the hospital roof. Meanwhile I had a dozen of our fellows down with fever and for the moment nowhere to send them. I took over in the afternoon and arranged things a bit, sent a party out in the town to commandeer pots and pans, china and lamps, and waited till next day, when I carried over all my stuff [medical]. Meanwhile I sent at once to work to clean up the centre of Es Salt and buried the horses and Turks, doing some of the digging myself to encourage the others, cleaned up the stream as it ran through our camp, and later buried everything for two and a half miles below Salt and two miles above – in all about sixty horses, twenty Turks and twenty other oddments. Next day I

> got to work on the hospital and dressed the cases the Turkish ones not touched for six days were awfully foul – and I got things comfortable. Next day the Welsh Ambulance came and took over the hospital and my work.[32]

During the next day, 1 May, as already noted the 4th Australian Light Horse Brigade was fighting at Damiye, where guns and vehicles were lost to the enemy and personnel of the Light Horse Field Ambulance were taken captive by the enemy. The unit was then reinforced by the 5th Mounted Field Ambulance. The Australian Mounted Division Collecting Station, which had been under command of the ADMS ANZAC Division, was ordered to move to the junction of the main road with Wadi Abu Muhair.

Throughout the day 372 casualties were admitted to and evacuated from this station without any difficulty.

During 2 May the situation at Shunet Nimrin remained unchanged. At the same time the cavalry units in the hills were fighting superior enemy forces and their situation was becoming difficult. The field ambulances in the Es Salt area ran short of dressings, anti-tetanic serum, chloroform, sutures, and medical comforts, which were supplied in two ways. The first was a donkey ammunition convoy which had managed to climb the difficult track from Umm Shert during the night. The other way was more interesting and, to some extent, an innovation.

When the Desert Mounted Corps HQ was assigned command of the second raid, Colonel Rupert Downes, the Corps DDMS, assumed responsibility for the medical side of the operation. Being very resourceful and, as General H. Chauvel, commander of the Desert Mounted Corps, defined him, 'one that loved soldiering second only to medicine,'[33] Colonel Downes had planned beforehand a drop of medical supplies from an airplane. Planning was not simple because neither Colonel Downes nor any of the officers fighting in Palestine had any experience with air supply. Due to the short time allotted to preparations for the raid, no preliminary trials could be carried out. The only experience acquired on the entire Turkish front at the time was that which had been gained during the siege of Kut el Amara in Mesopotamia at the beginning of 1916.

Colonel Downes and the pilots decided to act according to the experience gained there, even though they had only theoretical knowledge of it. The medical supplies were packed into motor car tires and wrapped with sandbags, while bottles and vials were wrapped carefully in cotton-wool. Forty pounds of medical supplies had been prepared in this manner in Jerusalem, from where the airplanes took off. The tires were dropped from a height of 1,000 feet and reached the intended unit. Unfortunately, most of the vials and bottles containing medications and chloroform were broken. The air-drop of medical supplies was a unique episode in the medical history of the Palestine campaign.[34]

On 3 May the enemy continued to press the cavalry brigades so hard that their situation became critical. As already related, the C-in-C ordered a withdrawal from Es Salt, a decision that raised the problem of medical evacuation from the Es Salt area. Until then only forty-two slightly wounded soldiers had been evacuated on horseback. There were many with severe injuries being treated at the advanced dressing station located in a Greek Orthodox church in Es Salt. Some of the wounded had been at the station for almost three days. Most of these casualties could not ride and the available twenty-nine *cacolet* camels, together with several horses which had lost their riders, were not enough for their evacuation. It was through efficient arrangements that all casualties were evacuated: anyone who could ride, even though severely wounded, was allowed to do so while all the rest were loaded into *cacolet*s and on camel-back. Only two mortally wounded soldiers who could not be moved were left to die at the station.

The camel convoy left Es Salt by 1930, the casualties escorted by the personnel of the advanced dressing station. The convoy made its way under – fortunately inefficient – fire from local irregulars. The night descent to Umm Shert was a long and dangerous march, the wounded suffering terribly. When the voyage was over, two men were found dead in their *cacolet*s. The convoy eventually reached the Australian Mounted Division Collecting Station at the Wadi Abu Muhair junction from where, after being fed and dressed, the wounded soldiers were evacuated by ambulances to the ANZAC Mounted Division Receiving Station. Further evacuation took place to the Corps Main Dressing Station at Jericho. Eighty-one casualties underwent surgery at the Desert Mounted Corps Operating Unit of the MDS. All the operations were for urgent situations, twenty-three of them for chest, abdominal, and pelvic wounds. Only six of those operated upon died.

During the raid 1,076 wounded and 708 sick were admitted to the main dressing station at Jericho. The majority were evacuated to the casualty clearing stations in Jerusalem without any further problems.

> Arrangements were now put in hand to evacuate the wounded and such of the camel transport as was not required with the fighting troops, down the El Shert track, preparatory to the withdrawal of the whole force. [...] What the wounded men in the cacolet must have suffered during this terrible journey can scarcely be imagined. It was past mid-day before the last camel had cleared Es Salt.[35]

When General Chauvel, who commanded the raid, tried to apologize to General Allenby for what he considered to be a failure, especially for the loss of guns, the C-in-C would not listen: 'Failure be damned' was his response.[36] For a far-sighted commander such as General Allenby, the raid had served its strategic goals.

> From the military point of view, this remarkable raid, though tactically a failure, served a strategic purpose of great importance by holding east of the Jordan quite one third of the whole Turkish force.[37]
>
> The raid was to have in the months to come a very important effect: to concentrate the attention of the enemy command on the Jordan Valley, and thereby to assist materially the final British offensive.[38]

However, from the medical point of view, the results were different: the failure to retain a hold in the hills beyond the Jordan condemned the mounted troops to bivouac during the summer in the Jordan Valley with all its hazards to the health of the troops.

7

A DIFFERENT BATTLE: THE ANTI-MALARIA CAMPAIGN, SUMMER 1918

'Every man in the force was made to feel some personal responsibility in the fight against the pest.'

Acting Sgt. James Eneas Scott, 2nd London Sanitary Company, RAMC (IWM, Document 79/1/1)

The failure of the second attempt to occupy the high ground around Es Salt made it imperative that EEF troops should hold a future line in the Jordan Valley. This was the right decision from the military point of view, as it took into consideration several factors. The first was the enemy's ability to attack the British eastern flank at very short notice. Secondly, it took into account the immediate and future plans of Sheikh Feisal's Arab army. But the third factor was probably the most important: it supported General Allenby's plans for the final offensive against the Turkish army. This future campaign could not be mounted before the autumn due to considerations related to the situation on the Western Front. A large-scale battle had been raging since March in that main theatre of the war. Some of the most experienced infantry units had already been transferred from Palestine to Europe and were replaced by inexperienced Indian cavalry and infantry units. What this entailed for the C-in-C EEF was that he had to deploy his units along the various front lines in the most economical manner. The practical implication was that units of considerable size would be spending the hot season in an area where 'no European had passed a summer.'[1]

The southern Jordan Valley was the middle zone of a wider plain, more than ten miles wide and almost 1,300 feet below sea level, bounded on both sides by steep mountains reaching the height of 2,700 feet above sea level. It thus had the form of a deep bath. It was known to be an extremely hot area where summer temperatures might reach more than 120°F. In this area, where most of the troops would be stationed, the average summer temperatures were about 110°F.

> It was decided that the Jordan Valley had to be occupied to make possible the autumn campaign which was being planned. It was generally accepted that no White man had ever before lived through a summer there, and even the flies died in the heat. […] The Turk cheered us up by dropping leaflets telling us: 'In August flies die; in September men die and we will be coming to bury you in October.'[2]

One of the troopers would write in his memoirs:

> In this climate and under such conditions, His Majesty's troops, white, brown, and black, held the line throughout the summer of 1918, and it is safe to say that few other troops in the Great War endured greater hardships and discomfort than did the Jordan Valley force.[3]

Another health problem in the Jordan Valley during the summer was the dust. Powdery in nature, it was created by any movement of a car or an animal, remained in the air for long hours, and made breathing and seeing difficult. In addition to the heat and the severe humidity, caused by the extreme evaporation of the Dead Sea water due to the heat, the dust made life in the area unbearable. Flies, scorpions, poisonous snakes, and other pests were the only creatures inhabiting the valley.

Under these conditions, almost every scratch became infected. General Allenby, who frequently visited the units in the Jordan Valley, did not like the sight of Australians riding in shorts – he considered this both unmilitary and risky for the soldiers' health. He therefore issued an order forbidding troops to ride in shorts, which became a source of dispute, as the soldiers ignored it. Eventually, a compromise was reached when Allenby agreed that soldiers may ride in long slacks of Khaki drill.[4]

However, the worst health problem awaiting the troops intending to bivouac in the area was malaria, endemic and very prevalent. Malaria in Palestine manifested itself clinically either in the benign tertian form or the malignant subtertian form. While the benign form of malaria, caused by Plasmodium vivax, was mainly a severe relapsing febrile disease which neutralized its victims to a large extent, the malignant form caused by Plasmodium falciparum was not only severe, but also lethal in some cases. Various species of the Anopheles mosquito were the vectors of the disease, transmitting the plasmodia from one infected human being to another by their bite. Anopheline mosquitoes were particularly prevalent in the Jordan Valley and in the Sharon Plain, along the Mediterranean coast north of Jaffa.[5]

One can easily imagine the detrimental effect of this disease on any military organization and its ability to function. Palestine was not the only front where malaria was prevalent. At the time of the Palestine campaigns it affected severely the British army units in East Africa. It was one of the diseases prevalent in Mesopotamia and also in Macedonia.

General Milne, the C-in-C in Macedonia, stated in a despatch that during the spring of 1917 British offensive initiatives had to be cancelled on his front due to huge losses of manpower caused by malaria. 'It can hardly be doubted that the operations throughout have been hampered by the high rates of sickness,' he wrote.[6] In fact, it was even worse: not only did any offence initiative have to be abandoned, malaria also forced the army in the Struma Valley to retreat to a new line to avoid being devastated by the disease.[7]

The troops feared malaria; their attitude might be reflected in the writings of individual soldiers:

> Gunshot wounds take their toll, but mostly it is the malaria; many would willingly have wounds in exchange for this cursed fever. It brings about a seesawing temperature. One minute its victims are sweating with heat, the next rolled shivering in blankets, shivering when the shade temperature is one hundred and twenty or more. Often the blood turns jet black, they cannot eat, just lie in the shade doing nothing but drink huge quantities of water. It is not possible for everyone developing fever to be removed, as this would mean the line becoming deserted; only the very bad cases go out.[8]

Similar reflections on malaria even were even expressed in poetry:

You, with your winding creeping course,
What of the men of our Southern Horse?
Valley of night, with your winged pest,
What of our heroes now at rest,
    Down by your Dead, salt Sea?
What of the ones we have left behind?
What of these men of our kith and Kind,
Nigh where your blood stream hiss?
Better the true and unerring shot!
Better the Death when their blood runs hot –
Than this,
    Malaria! Malaria!

You, with your aged river's flow,
What of our Riders laid below?
Valley of Death, with your torpid heat,
Look where your swirling hill streams meet,
    Down by your Dead, salt Sea!
Look to the ones on your mounded knoll!
Look to the ones of your chosen toll!
Those of your fevered kiss!
Better the blast of the rending shell!
Better the toll of the War God's knell,
Than this,
    Malaria! Malaria![9]

General Allenby was aware of the problem posed by malaria from the various reports he was receiving as well as from his deep knowledge of history.

> It was typical to General Allenby going one day in the neighbourhood of Ludd, he drifted into a bacteriological laboratory where he saw some charts on the wall and asked for their meaning. 'Well Sir' said the bacteriologist, 'those are charts of the seasonal incidence of malignant malaria in the Plain of Sharon, and I think this is the reason why Richard Coeur de Lion never got to Jerusalem. His army was nearly

> destroyed by fever, and I find that he came down the coast in September, when malignant malaria was at its height.' This sort of information was manna from heaven to Allenby, and he never forgot it.[10]

Data concerning malaria in Palestine, of which the British authorities were aware, had already been collected by German scientists of the 'International Hygiene Bureau' in 1912–13. According to these data an annual epidemic of malignant malaria had hit Palestine during the autumn months, its peak being mid-October, while the benign malaria was at its height during the summer.[11] However, there were no data concerning malaria in the Jordan Valley, as this area had never been investigated.

Colonel Richard H. Luce, at the time the DDMS XX Corps and later DMS EEF, recalled:

> As regards to malaria we started with very little knowledge about the prevalence of the disease in this part of the country which had been little frequented by tourists and travellers. We knew, however, that parts of central and northern Palestine had a very evil reputation in the summer and the autumn months.[12]

Lt-General Harry Chauvel, commander of the Desert Mounted Corps, remembered that 'we were concerned about the spread of malaria, especially if the Corps were to fight in the Jordan Valley, and there had been conferences on the subject long before the fall of Jerusalem.'[13] However, information concerning the prevalence of the disease in the Jordan Valley was very scarce.

General Allenby's attitude towards health hazards in Palestine was the keystone of the policy created by his staff, as manifested in the unprecedented support of the medical services in their fight against malaria.[14] In his memoirs, Surgeon General Luce recalled how the decision to remain in the Jordan Valley during the summer was taken, together with its various implications:

> The problem confronting him [General Allenby] at the beginning of 1918 was this: you are holding a line across a country which is known to be intensely malarious. Parts of it, for example the Jordan Valley and the Plain of Sharon near the

> sea, are uninhabitable for Europeans during the late summer and autumn. If these areas are held during these periods without very active measures to deal with malaria, your army will be decimated with the disease. It was a great problem. He decided that he must hold the line, but he did not send his sanitary officers to the base. He trusted them and gave them a free hand – a great decision and characteristic of the man.[15]

The troops to be selected to hold the line in the Jordan Valley would have several duties, mainly patrolling during the nights and building the new fortified line by digging and wiring during the days. Such a work regime would no doubt deprive the troops of the ability to rest and sleep properly. To all these would be added the continuous toil of the anti-malaria campaign.

When General Allenby decided to hold the Jordan Valley during the summer, his policy was to expose as few troops as possible to the threats of that area. This meant that the troops chosen for the mission should be those best able to endure the summer in the Jordan Valley while executing all their planned duties and be capable of fighting the enemy at any moment. The C-in-C came to the conclusion that the line should be held by a mobile mounted force, and his choice fell upon the ANZAC units. Later in the summer, when the newly arrived Indian cavalry units would be capable of sharing in the tasks and duties of the Jordan Valley line, they should replace the Australian troops. Thus, every division would undergo a tour of duty in the Jordan Valley for four to six weeks, after which they were sent for convalescence at 'Rest Stations.'

The concept of 'Rest Stations' was not created during the spring and summer of 1918. Already in 1917, while the ANZACs had been stationed in the Sinai Desert, their ADMS, Lt-Colonel Rupert Downes, felt the need for such stations. The main reason then was the state of many weary soldiers who had been suffering from gastrointestinal ailments as well as from 'desert sores.'[16] Colonel Downes realized that what these soldiers really needed was just a place where they could rest, eat, maintain personal hygiene, and sleep properly. Colonel Downes' Rest Stations, especially those near the Mediterranean seashore, had proved a great success: not only did the soldiers enjoy their stay, but they had not been lost to their units. During the spring of 1918 such stations were established near the Mediterranean coast and in a monastery in Jerusalem, where the soldiers could rest from their Jordan

Valley experience. They were staffed by the personnel of the tent-immobile subdivisions of field ambulances.

The anti-malaria campaign conducted during the spring and summer of 1918 was based on the ability to diagnose the disease accurately and rapidly, on an understanding of the mosquito's life cycle, on the thorough knowledge of the areas in which the risk of malaria was high, and on the commanders' support at all levels.[17] Major-General Swan, DMS EEF, appointed Major A.E. Austen, an entomologist from the British Museum, as special adviser for the anti-malaria campaign, whose plan was developed under his guidance. The actual efforts in the field to eradicate mosquito breeding were supervised by the administrative officers of the divisions, with the professional backing of the divisional sanitary sections. This meant that, like any other military operation, the unit commander was responsible for the anti-malaria campaign. Due to General Allenby's unique attitude towards prevention of disease, it was not perceived as a 'health issue' concerning the medical service alone. Thus 'every man in the force was made to feel some personal responsibility in the fight against the pest.'[18]

The Regimental Medical Officers were instructed how to deal with suspected cases of malaria. Blood smears from suspected individuals should be taken and sent to the nearest 'Malarial Diagnosis Station.' When the disease was positively diagnosed, treatment should begin as soon as possible, mainly at the hospital level, and this for two different reasons. The first, obviously, was for the patient's sake: early initiation of treatment reduced the risk of clinical complications, mainly in cases of the malignant form of the disease.[19] The second reason was for the benefit of the unit: to reduce the number of infected soldiers whose blood stream was a source of plasmodia and eventually for the further spread of infection by mosquitoes.

There were six Malarial Diagnosis Stations, each consisting of a specially trained medical officer and two orderlies who had also been trained in malarial diagnosis. All 'Station' teams, supplied with two microscopes and staining equipment, could diagnose the disease quickly and accurately in the field. The 'Stations' were backed up professionally by three 'Military Laboratories,' well equipped microbiological laboratories whose personnel consisted of bacteriologists as well as pathologists and other professionals who could respond to any health problem among the troops. Military Laboratory No. 2 was located at Lydda to deal with health problems among the XXI Corps units; Military Laboratory No. 3 was located at Jerusalem for the units of the

XX Corps, and the ANZAC Military Laboratory was established at Jericho and served the Desert Mounted Corps.

Every brigade has its 'Brigade malarial officer' whose responsibility it was to train the regimental anti-malarial squads. There were six to thirteen squads in every regiment, their main task being to locate potential mosquito breeding grounds. The outcome of the squads' work was a map of the whole area which enabled the ADMS and the divisional sanitary sections to plan the anti-mosquito action in the field.

Protecting soldiers from mosquito bites by specially designed gloves, hats, and garments seemed very unpractical. Anti-mosquito-nets were lacking and since most military activity took place during the night, their usefulness was doubtful in any case. The various repellents and ointments were found to be only partially helpful.[20]

The value of quinine as a prophylactic medication against malaria had been the subject of much debate and confusion before the war. Those who believed in its prophylactic value could not agree upon its proper dose. There was also no consensus concerning the value of quinine in the prevention of relapses of the disease. Based mainly on the Macedonian experience during the Great War, the general opinion did not support the use of quinine as a prophylactic. The practical outcome was that 'quinine prophylaxis was not employed by compulsion, though units wishing to do so, were given facilities to do so.'[21]

There was also disagreement among malaria experts considering the treatment of the first acute phase of the disease, i.e., whether quinine should be injected intravenously or in a deep injection into the gluteal muscles. In addition, the question of maintenance treatment to prevent future relapses of the disease was raised from time to time.[22] Thus, only the annihilation of the mosquitoes could efficiently prevent their bites and hence the transmission of the disease. The only way to achieve this efficiently was by controlling their breeding. An understanding of the mosquito life cycle was vital for planning the anti-malaria campaign. In order to breed, the Anopheline mosquitoes need standing clear water. This meant that the water of the rapidly flowing River Jordan did not pose a problem. However, its tributaries, which were surrounded by reeds and weeds and along which were located ponds, marshes, and swamps, were ideal breeding grounds for malaria transmitting mosquitoes. Other breeding places were irrigation canals, wells, and holes in the ground. After the initial survey of the area,

Major Austen defined the Jordan Valley as 'by far the worst I have seen either in Palestine or Macedonia.'[23]

The anti-malaria campaign included the clearing of reeds and weeds from all the tributaries of the Jordan and of the other streams in the area and also canalization and drainage of ponds and marshes. The work was carried out by soldiers reinforced by thousands of civilian labourers from the Egyptian Labour Corps who worked only where enemy shelling was unlikely. The work was efficient and thorough and all its goals were achieved. Then came the phase of supervision and maintenance whose objectives were detection of any signs of a new breeding ground so as to destroy it and maintenance of the already cleaned streams and canals.[24]

In the Sharon Plain, the western flank of the British forces, where the XXI Corps was holding the line along the Auja River, malaria was as prevalent as in the Jordan Valley. The two areas differed mainly in climatic conditions, those in the Sharon Plain being much more benign. The anti-malaria campaign in the Sharon Plain was organized along the same lines as in the Jordan Valley. Here the main problem was the Auja River itself, whose banks were cleared of all plants and weeds. Several units were assigned to clear the river and its tributaries. In the Sharon Plain rivers, streams, and irrigation canals were not the only source of mosquito breeding; wells and shell holes also had to be dealt with. While holes and pools were filled with sand, the wells were either sealed or had oil poured into them. Floating on the water, the oil prevented breeding but allowed the continued drawing of water from the well. Out of use wells were sealed. As in the Jordan Valley, an important phase in the campaign against malaria was the second one: supervision and maintenance of the previously cleaned potential breeding grounds. Oiling the wells, for example, had to be repeated every seven days during the whole season.[25] 'At Latron the great stunt was Pipe's anti-malaria work, carried for six and a quarter miles along the bed of that stream, consisting of the demolition of all vegetation from all the stream banks, cleaning and re-channeling the stream and bi-weekly oiling of all water.'[26]

On 18 April 1918 the DDMS XXI Corps, Colonel C.J. Macdonald, was transferred to Cairo to become ADMS 2nd Echelon at GHQ. He was replaced by Colonel E.P. Sewell, ADMS of the 74th Division, who took the anti-malaria campaign very seriously.

It might be interesting to once again cite Surgeon General Luce. Though quite ignoring the historical differences between the two epochs to which he referred and the developments and changes that had occurred in warfare techniques and military organization, one may still sense in Luce's comments both criticism towards former commanders' attitudes and at the same time his admiration of General Allenby's attitude to prevention of disease.

> It is not so many years since one of our greatest generals, Lord Wolsley wrote: 'The sanitary officer is the creation of recent years and as a general rule he is a very useless functionary. In the numerous campaigns where I have served with a sanitary officer, I can conscientiously state I have never known him make any useful suggestions, where as I have known him make many silly ones. It is not his fault, for with an army moving it is impossible to drain a town, as I have know suggested, or carry out any other great sanitary measures. […] In the future, as long as this fad continues, my recommendation is to leave him at the base, where he may find some useful occupation as a member of the Sanitary Board, which I think should have charge of all sanitary arrangements at the base.' I wonder how Lord Wolsley would have faced the proposition put before General Allenby in Palestine. Fortunately General Allenby was of a more open mind and belonged to a more enlightened age.[27]

The anti-malaria campaign in Palestine, which lasted all together for about six months, consumed about 222,840 man-days.[28]

General Allenby was personally involved in the anti-malaria campaign and was familiar with its details, just as in all his other campaigns. This may be demonstrated by his letter to General Wilson, the CIGS, in June 1918:

> I am campaigning against mosquitoes; draining, clearing, burning, etc; and hope, in a week or two, to have improved things. Many acres of bog have already been drained and cleared, and the drains, though some are as salt as the Dead Sea, and stink of sulphur, swarm with little, active fish. These will, I hope, feed on the larvae.[29]

Despite the anti-malaria work in the Jordan Valley, new cases of the disease were diagnosed every day. About 2 percent of the troops stationed in the Jordan Valley were evacuated to hospitals every week suffering from malaria.

It seemed as if the tremendous effort had been in vain, as testified by one of the soldiers of Chaytor's Force, stationed in the Jordan Valley: 'The malaria scourge has become so great that we struggle to decrease the mosquito pest, which is filling the hospitals to overflowing. Weeks of backbreaking toil in the grueling heat, many dropping as the fever grips them whilst they work [...].'[30] However, this soldier was mistaken, for most of these new cases were soldiers who had engaged in military activities either in No Man's Land or near the front lines. In both cases they had been exposed to the bites of mosquitoes which bred in enemy territory where no anti-malaria campaign had been undertaken. It was noted that the incidence of malaria among soldiers in rear units, where all anti-malaria measures had been taken, was much lower.

The anti-malaria campaign was indeed a success. In the XXI Corps, for example, the picture was quite clear: out of a force of roughly of 70,000 men only 7,271 cases of malaria were detected during a twenty-one-week period, of which 1,965 were cases of relapse rather than fresh ones. This meant that there were only 5,306 new cases, less than 7.6 percent of the force.

Thus, General Allenby was right when a year later he commented that 'the medical services combated malaria, the chief scourge of Syria and Palestine, with excellent results.'[31] This situation was about to change very shortly.

8

THE BATTLE OF MEGIDDO: THE LAST OFFENSIVE

'He told me that he realized before the Battle of Meggido that his danger was malaria.'

Sir James Barrett, 'The Halford Oration,' *Medical Journal of Australia* (1932) part II: 707–18.

'The work of the medical staff and ambulances during these arduous marches was performed with that unobtrusive efficiency to which we have become so accustomed that, because it is carried on behind the combatant line and therefore out of sight, we generally pass unnoticed.'

General G. de S. Barrow [OC the 4th Cavalry Division], *The Fire of Life* (London: Hutchinson, 1942), 214.

A year had passed since General Allenby assumed command of the EEF. During that year the EEF won the Third Battle of Gaza and captured southern Palestine, including Jerusalem. Though the victory at Gaza and the capture of Jerusalem – the Holy City – had some political and moral significance, these events did not bear any strategic impact on the total war in which Britain was engaged. The Palestine campaign was still considered a 'side show' by many.

In March 1917 General Maude had captured Baghdad and practically driven the Turkish army out of most of Mesopotamia. However, as in the case of Palestine, this military success, though it boosted British morale, did not have any strategic impact on the main theatre – the Western Front in Europe.

Both the War Office and General Allenby realized that only a complete victory over the Turkish army in Palestine, one that would prevent the Turkish forces from fighting in the future, had any substantial strategic value and justification. Allenby thought such a victory was possible but demanded some reinforcements in order to secure it. No reinforcements could be sent to the Middle East, for in March 1918 the German spring 'Ludendorff Offensive' was launched and the War Office ordered General Allenby to immediately send several of the EEF infantry divisions to the Western Front. The gap in manpower was gradually filled by Indian units which generally lacked previous combat experience. Thus, any attempt to resume an offensive in the near future was out of the question.

The main task facing the EEF during the spring and summer of 1918 was to train the new units and reorganize the remaining depleted divisions to prepare them for battle when the moment came. Luckily, due to the nature of the battlefields at the Western Front, there was no need for more cavalry units in that arena. Thus, the original two mounted divisions remained in Palestine while two other newly formed mounted divisions, based on the Indian 4th and 5th Cavalry Divisions, were added to the EEF. The 10th, 53rd, 54th, 60th, and 75th Divisions, which had been depleted of most of their infantry battalions, were augmented by new Indian battalions. Two Indian Infantry Divisions, the 3rd (Lahore) and the 7th (Meerut), were added to the XXI Corps. The ANZAC Mounted Division was augmented by the 20th Indian Brigade.

The new divisions arrived with their field ambulances. Though several field ambulances were short of personnel, it was thought that they could perform according to professional expectations.[1] EEF HQ, however, felt that increased hospital accommodation was needed for the arriving Indian divisions. General Allenby therefore demanded more hospitals, and six Indian General Hospitals were sent to Egypt from India and Mesopotamia. Five of them were placed on the Palestine L-of-C and one was established at Suez.[2]

During July 1918 the German spring offensive on the Western Front came to a halt without gaining any real achievement. With the military situation in Europe again becoming stalemated, the option of an offensive in the

Middle East was once more discussed. It was the right time to decide about the objectives and feasibility of a future offensive. Already in late December 1917 the War Office had estimated the cost in manpower of an operation aimed at capturing northern Palestine up to the sources of the River Jordan to be about 57,000 casualties and probably about 20,000 sick soldiers.[3] If these figures were correct, the conclusion was that in order to resume operations on a large scale, some reinforcements should be sent to Palestine.

These earlier estimates, however, were no longer relevant, as the situation had changed entirely. The Turkish army in the summer of 1918 was not the same as it had been during the summer of 1917. It had lost much of its confidence; many soldiers were deserting every day, and the outcome was severe lack of manpower in the majority of the units. Many soldiers had health problems, mainly gastrointestinal and deficiency diseases. The Turkish army as a whole suffered from a shortage of supplies. Yet, a new Supreme Commander was appointed to the Turkish forces in Syria and Palestine: German General Otto Liman von Sanders, who replaced General Falkenhayn on 1 March 1918. Liman von Sanders brought with him several capable and experienced staff officers, both Turkish and German. He himself came with the reputation of the defeat he had inflicted upon the British forces in Gallipoli.[4] The force he now commanded was still a formidable enemy, especially when it was on the defence.

The Turkish army was now organized in three armies, two to the west of the Jordan and one to its east, holding a lengthy defensive line from the Mediterranean coast in the Sharon Plain in the west, through the mountains of Samaria to the Jordan Valley in the east. The two armies stationed west of the Jordan, the VIII and the VII, consisted altogether of 17,000 infantry soldiers. The IV army in the Jordan Valley and beyond the Jordan had the vital task of protecting the Hejaz railway. It consisted of 6,000 infantry and about 2,000 cavalry troops. Liman's headquarters were in Nazareth.

The EEF at that time numbered some 57,000 infantry soldiers organized in seven infantry divisions and 12,000 mounted troops in four cavalry divisions. It also had 540 guns, 100 of them being medium and heavy artillery. Thus, the EEF was significantly superior both in men and artillery over its Ottoman opponent. It was specifically superior both in the number and quality of mounted troops. It also held the upper hand in logistics, for during the first months of 1918 the railway from Egypt to Palestine had been doubled and 2,000 tons of supplies were transported daily by train to the EEF troops.

During the third battle of Gaza the Turkish army, though sustaining many casualties and losing the whole front line from Beersheba to Gaza, managed to beat an orderly retreat, maintaining its formations and establishing new lines of defence. This meant that though the objective of capturing Gaza was fully achieved, the British victory had not been decisive. Another incomplete victory was considered unacceptable this time.

General Allenby's basic plan for the destruction of the Turkish army was quite simple: to break through the Turkish defences with his infantry and thus enable the superior cavalry forces to advance rapidly to the enemy's rear. There it would cut the Turkish lines of communication and prevent any attempt at an organized retreat. Allenby intended to surprise the enemy and this was indeed achieved by various methods of deception and diversion. Deception was both strategic and tactical: when the offensive began, the Turkish command was taken completely by surprise as they had not expected any offensive at that time, definitely not along the coastal plain. To ensure the victory of the infantry it was planned to strike the Turkish defence line with a superior power of five infantry divisions along a narrow sector of eight miles from the seashore inland.[5]

The major operation was assigned to the XXI Corps whose attack would be preceded by a short but massive artillery barrage. The XX Corps, which comprised only two infantry divisions, would simultaneously attack in the hills to the north, its objective being the Nablus road. Chaytor's Force in the Jordan Valley would continue its demonstrations as part of the deception and diversion, in order to attract enemy forces to the east. It was planned that as the main offensive began in the coastal plain Chaytor's Force would seal the bridges over the Jordan to prevent any Turkish forces from retreating across the Jordan.

General Allenby's plan took shape in two stages. In the first he came to the conclusion that an offensive aimed at the destruction of the Turkish army was feasible using the EEF's own resources. However, the second stage was much more far-seeing: it was then he realized that by more daring use of the same infantry and cavalry forces which he intended to exploit, he could achieve a definite and decisive victory over the enemy. This understanding was the key to his final plan.

While Allenby's initial plan intended to destroy the Turkish army between the existing front line and the geographical line of Nahr Iskanderune–Tul Karm–Nablus–River Jordan, the objective of his final one was annihilation of the two Turkish armies in Palestine. According to the new plan, the Desert Mounted Corps' objective was not just to take Mesudie Junction and the mountain passes; it now became the strategic objective of capturing El Affule, the most important railway junction in northern Palestine. From this junction the western branch of the Hejaz railway led north to Haifa and south to Jenin-Nablus and Tul Karm. Capturing the El Affule Junction, expected on the second day of the offensive, together with the taking of Beisan in the Jordan Valley, south of the Lake of Galilee, meant complete encirclement of the retreating Turkish army. The XXI Corps, after accomplishing its task in the plain, would turn eastwards and together with the XX Corps would mount a pincer-like operation that would destroy the Turkish army west of the Jordan.

General Allenby also realized that time was one of the limiting factors of his plan. He was aware that his troops were to fight in enemy territory in which no anti-malaria activity had been conducted. This meant that when the forces, mainly the mounted units, would break through the enemy lines the troops would be bitten by the anopheles mosquitoes. The incubation period, before the actual clinical manifestations of the disease might appear, was expected to be between seven to fourteen days. Then many of the troops might manifest the clinical symptoms of the disease which might be severe and incapacitate many of them. He was also aware that at that time of the year the main form of malaria was the malignant one. After the war General Allenby told a senior physician that he was aware of the danger and made his plans accordingly: the decisive victory should be achieved during several days, before malaria struck.[6]

While the virtues of this final plan lay mainly in daring simplicity and clarity, its various medical implications were relatively complex. The medical plan, expected to provide professional solutions for all kinds of health and medical problems during the offensive, had to be creative and sophisticate indeed.[7] The medical planning was conducted in accordance and in pace with the operative plans. It was to become a comprehensive system serving the troops during a daring large-scale operation. Much thought and effort were invested at various medical levels. The DMS, Surgeon General Swan, was very instrumental in the planning and preparations for the offensive and cooperated in the most efficient way with the DDMSs of the three Corps. All divisional ADMSs participated in the various stages of planning and staff work.[8]

The medical plan devised by Major General Swan together with the corps DDMSs was based on several assumptions. A large number of casualties was to be expected during the fighting by the infantry divisions at the front line. In a case of extremely hard fighting during the first stage of the offensive, or in a situation in which the infantry had failed to break through the front line at the first attempt, the evacuation of casualties from the front line to the medical echelons might be very tedious. Medical units were to support any combat unit fighting in a defined zone and would not be committed solely to their own brigades. Cooperation among medical units might at some time be very important; however, it would depend on meticulous planning and coordination at the battlefield level. Due to expected difficulties in evacuation, the advanced surgical units should be located close to the front line. Special routes should be set aside solely for medical evacuation. In sectors where roads were scarce or of poor quality, wire roads should be prepared to allow proper medical evacuation. Shortage of water might be a problem during the offensive, an issue that should be tackled and solved before it arose.

Assuming that the assault would proceed as planned, it would lead to the collapse of the Turkish army. The outcome might be that many wounded or sick Turkish soldiers might reach EEF medical facilities. Their number might be enormous, and precautions should be taken so as not to be overwhelmed by these prisoners of war. The prisoners might suffer from epidemic and infectious diseases; they should be diagnosed and treated properly but at the same time isolated, in order not to transmit diseases to EEF troops. To cope with all these problems, several Detention Hospitals had been brought to various locations before the offensive actually began: No. 2 Egyptian Detention Hospital was located at Lydda, while No. 4 Egyptian Detention Hospital was located at Wilhelma.[9]

At the beginning of September the DMS EEF issued an order concerning the prevention of malaria. Every soldier was to receive ten grains of quinine daily as a prophylactic treatment against malaria.[10] All Medical Officers must be aware of the possibility of an outbreak of malaria among the troops.

During the first phase of the assault, the XXI Corps, comprising five infantry divisions and one cavalry brigade, was to get the lion's share of the offensive – and most probably also of the casualties. The corps' task was to attack and capture the enemy lines of defence along a front of eight miles from the sea eastwards. Its plan also included the establishment of bridgeheads beyond Nahr el Falik, which would allow the mounted forces to quickly advance to the enemy's rear. When this stage was accomplished, the whole corps would use its most easterly division, the 54th, as a pivot and swing eastwards. The 54th Division would then attack the enemy in the area of Kefar Kasim; the 3rd Division would attack at Kefar Saba and then move on to Qalqilye and Jiljulie. The 75th Division would attack at Et Tire together with the 7th, which would then continue to Taiybe and Falamie. The hardest task was that of the 60th Division, the most westerly division of the corps: after establishing a bridgehead beyond Nahr el Falik it would turn eastwards and march to Tul Karm, in order to capture the town itself and cut the Tul Karm–Nablus road and the railway east of Tul Karm.

The medical support for the XXI Corps offensive included various medical units. Advanced dressing stations would be located at the 'heads' of the wire roads, which were prepared at the last moment to maintain strict secrecy. Every division was instructed by the DDMS to open only one main dressing station during the initial stage of the battle. Taking into account that five divisions would attack simultaneously along a relatively small front, the usual mode of organization was altered: four field ambulances, operating at the western side of the front, were grouped in pairs: one pair for the 60th and the 7th Divisions and one pair for the 75th and the 3rd Divisions.

These potent medical bodies were established at specially constructed sidings on the light railway. The main dressing stations were to be located during the night of 18 September. The 54th Division, which would operate in the eastern sector in very rugged terrain, needed special medical arrangements. During the initial stage of the offensive it would establish an ADS at a quarry in Mejdel Yaba, and later on this ADS would be reinforced and become an MDS. Other sections of the 54th Division Field Ambulances were ordered to push on behind their brigades. Casualties were to be retained at the MDS until a road would reach it and then they would be evacuated by motor ambulance cars to Wilhelma Station. There would be established No. 15 Combined Clearing Hospital, an Advanced Operating Unit, and No. 4 Egyptian Detention Hospital. The medical facility at Wilhelma Station was near the Rantie railhead. Casualties could be further evacuated either by motor ambulance cars through specially provided wire roads to No. 33 Combined Clearing Hospital in Jaffa or by light train to Lydda, where two British, two Indian, and one French Casualty Clearing Stations were located together with two Egyptian Stationary Hospitals and a special hospital for prisoners of war.

Sketch 30.

MEGIDDO, 1918. Situation at Zero hour, 19th Sept., 1918.

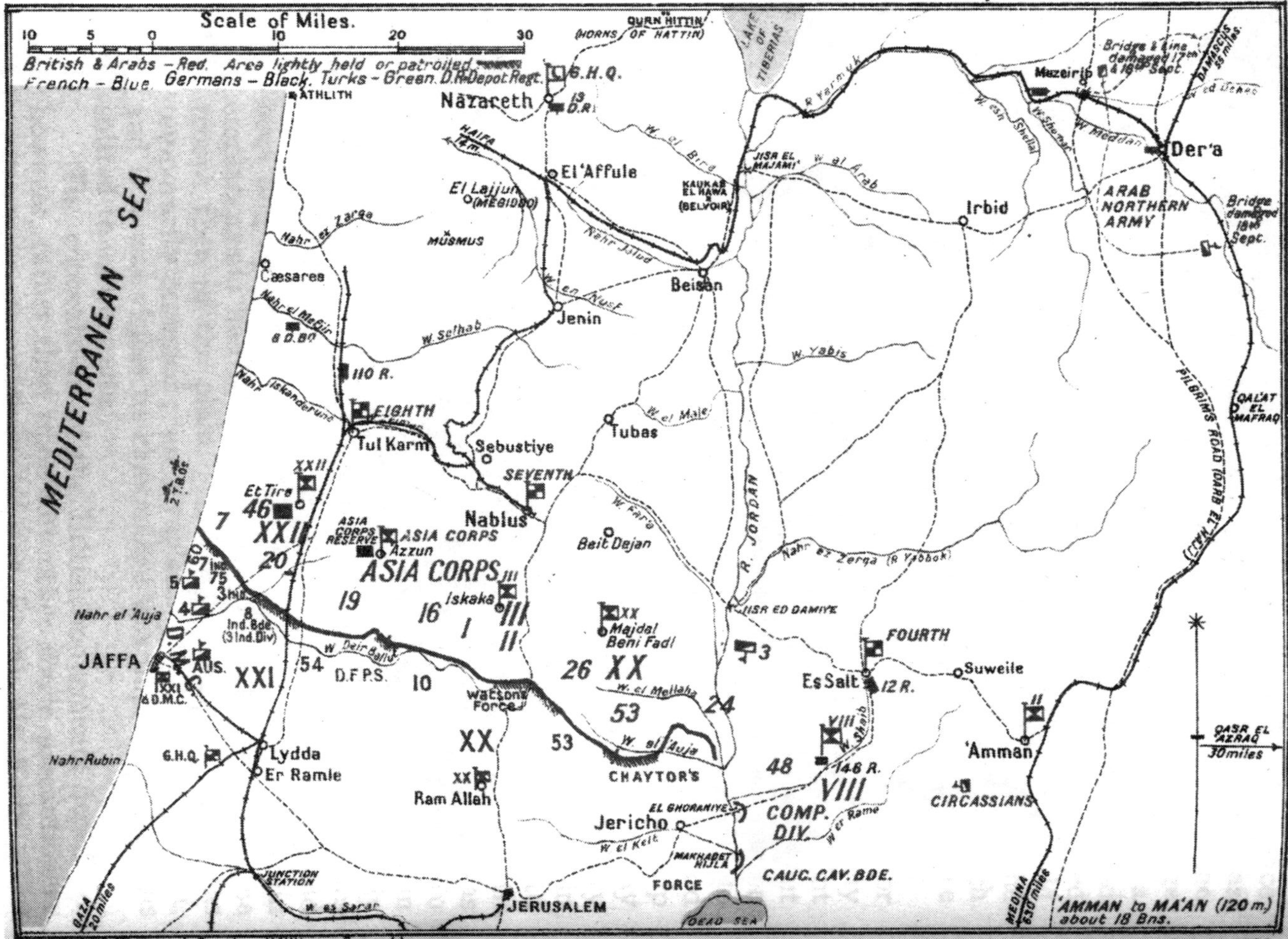

PLATE 48

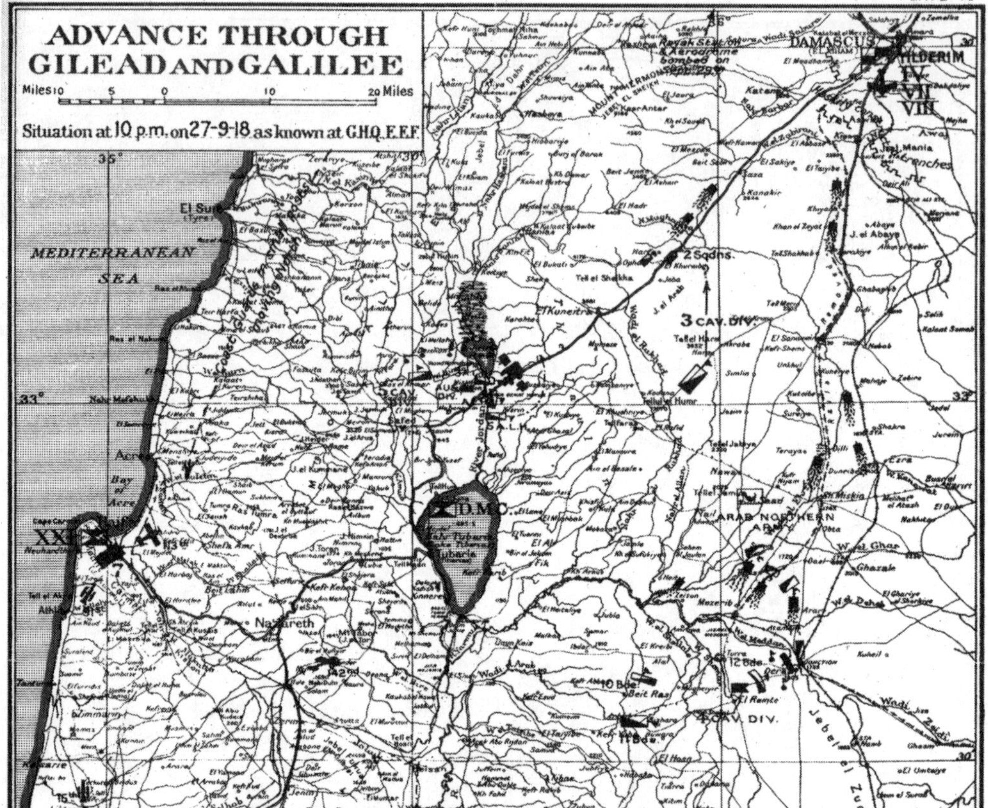

Printed by the Survey of Egypt, Dec. 1918 (0453)

Reprinted in England 1919.

The XXI corps was allotted 13 heavy and 106 light ambulances in addition to the ambulances that had already been in use by the divisions. Every field ambulance was allotted 50 camels for medical evacuation, 34 of which had the usual *cacolets*, the rest were supplied with 'poles and nets' stretchers which had been found more comfortable for sitting casualties.

The field ambulances of the four divisions other than the 54th, which would not be unpacked, were expected to join their divisions during the second phase of the offensive. Those of the 3rd Division would join it after the capture of Jiljulie and open there. One field ambulance of the 75th Division was planned to open a Rest Station at Qalqilie for casualties of various units of the corps coming in from the north and east. Another field ambulance of the same division was ready to open if necessary at Miske, southwest of Et Tire. The 7th Division reserve field ambulances were to follow the division to Et Tire and Taiybe. All field ambulances were instructed to evacuate their sick and wounded as rapidly as possible to enable joining their divisions by the nearest routes. Most of the field ambulances were expected to reach the Tuk Karm–Rantieh road and there to open for the treatment of casualties arriving during the second phase of the offensive.

If necessary, the 60th Division was to form a fresh Main Dressing Station at Nahr el Falik together with one of the field ambulances in reserve and to bring the others up with the troops to Tul Karm. Possible casualties beyond Nahr el Falik, including those of the mounted divisions, would be carried forward by ambulance to Tul Karm, from where they would be evacuated to No. 15 Casualty Clearing Hospital at Rantie.[11]

Special water columns, each consisting of 2,200 camels of the Camel Transport Corps, were prepared to carry 44,000 gallons of water for the corps troops. A water pipeline conveying water from Nahr el Auja to Jelil was constructed just before the concentration of the divisions took place.

Thus, the medical support plan for the offensive of the XXI Corps had several virtues. It maintained flexibility: at any given moment there were enough uncommitted medical units which could be utilized either in their own divisional sector or elsewhere. During the first phase of the attack, the infantry medical units, operating as dressing stations, were prepared to treat and evacuate all casualties. This allowed the cavalry medical units to move behind their brigades to the enemy's rear without loss of time. For the second phase, there were enough units in reserve which could be opened if needed.

As noted, the plan called for the Desert Mounted Corps units to rely on the medical services of the XXI Corps during the first phase of the offensive. After breaking through the enemy lines, a small number of casualties was expected who would be treated by the mobile sections of the cavalry field ambulances which would follow the mounted brigades and manage to keep up with them. During the second phase they were expected to evacuate casualties to Tul Karm and later on according to developments.[12]

The Corps' Advanced Operating Unit and two Malarial Diagnosis Stations were ordered to follow the 4th Cavalry division and the Australian Mounted Division. The Corps' heavy motor ambulance wagons were exchanged for light ones. The field ambulances were augmented with more camels for carrying a reserve supply of two days' rations and medical comforts for each Divisional MDS. 'Successful experiments were made in the use of motor tubes for dropping medical supplies and comforts from airplanes.'[13]

The XX Corps' plan was to attack the VII Army front lines and destroy them with two independent divisional forces and to advance to the Nablus road. The medical plan had to provide independent answers for the two divisions, up to the Nablus road line. Two MDSs would be established for the 53rd Division operating on the eastern flank of the corps, based on two of the divisional Combined Field Ambulances. Casualties would be retained at the MDSs until the Nablus road was reached and would be evacuated to the road by camel ambulance transport, from where they were to be transported by motor ambulance cars.

On the western flank, the operations theatre of the 10th Division, an MDS consisting of a Combined Field Ambulance and an Advanced Operating Unit would be located at Nebi Saleh. From there the casualties would be further evacuated to the rear by motor ambulance cars. Lightly wounded would be evacuated from El Lubban to Lydda by a light train, under the command of the ADMS 10th Division. Every division was instructed to hold one field ambulance in reserve for the last phase of the campaign – the battle for the town of Nablus. Collecting Stations were planned to be established at several points along the Nablus road during the advance of the troops to take care of lightly wounded stragglers. The DDMS assigned Colonel E.J.R. Evatt, formerly ADMS 53rd Division, to conduct and control medical evacuation in the corps' area.

For the casualties of the XX Corps and Chaytor's Force, who might be evacuated to Jerusalem, an evacuation route by train from Jerusalem to Lydda was arranged. Twelve trains were available daily for this mission, each comprising ten coaches that could accommodate 200 lying patients.[14]

It was decided to prefer forward evacuation of casualties, thus bringing them more speedily to a road where motor ambulances could be used. The decision was based on the lessons of previous battles where it had been found that evacuation in wagons or *cacolets* might be detrimental to the patients. 'Forward evacuation' meant an unusual medical system of evacuation. Usually it was the outcome of a situation on the battlefield in which casualties could not be evacuated to the rear. In such a scenario, the various sections of the field ambulances were prepared to care for the casualties and carry them on with them, in the direction of the advancing brigades. Casualties were retained by these units until they could be transferred to other medical units located in the area according to plan: either other units of the same division, which could not halt previously, or medical units of adjacent divisions that reached the advanced area from other directions.

The basic component of Chaytor's Force was the ANZAC Mounted Division which was reinforced by the 20th Indian Brigade and four infantry battalions. The force's medical units included the field ambulances of the ANZAC Mounted Division, the 1st Welsh Field Ambulance of the 53rd (Welsh) Division, two Indian field ambulances, the ANZAC Advanced Operating Unit with the ANZAC Field Laboratory, and a detachment from the 2nd Stationary Hospital which arrived from Egypt. For medical evacuation, the force was augmented by 60 *cacolet* camels from the 10th and 53rd Divisions of the XX Corps. Medical treatment and evacuation of battle casualties were planned to be identical to those used previously during the Amman and Es Salt raids. It was expected that at a later stage, when Chaytor's Force captured Es Salt and Amman, it would establish there MDSs based on the field ambulances of the ANZAC Mounted Division.

Two days before the offensive was launched, the DMS, Major-General William T. Swan had to be replaced. Colonel Richard H. Luce, DDMS of the XX Corps, was appointed his successor. Colonel Luce had been with the British forces in the Mediterranean from the beginning of the war, including the Dardanelles operations, the battles of Gaza, and the raids across the Jordan. He was considered by his superiors, as well as by his peers, a very capable medical officer. Colonel Luce was succeeded as DDMS XX Corps by Colonel E.B. Dowsett, the ADMS of the 60th Division. By that time all preparations were in their final stage, and the new DMS was familiar with all the medical plans for the offensive. Thus, medical organization for the offensive was not affected by the change. However, it was an unusual affair which passed quite unnoticed in later written histories.

Only the background of the event was briefly mentioned in the official history of the 60th Division, and no explanation provided: 'On August 22nd, Lieutenant-Colonel Bridges, D.S.O., commanding the 179th Indian Combined Ambulance, was unfortunately drowned whilst bathing at Jaffa, being on a visit to G.H.Q.'[15] Lt-Col. J.J. Abraham, the ADMS of Palestine L-of-C, referred to the unusual case of the dismissal of General Swan in his diary:

> I was in daily contact with the DMS, Major General Swan, whose office was at GHQ, Bir Salim, two miles away from Ramleh. Everything seemed to be going smoothly. And then one afternoon I had a message that the DMS and his acting ADMS, Lieutenant-Colonel Bridges, had gone to Jaffa for a swim, and that Bridges had been drowned and the DMS rescued with some difficulty. This was most distressing. [...]
>
> The main trouble, however, was the General. The death of Bridges upset him very much. He just went to pieces for a fortnight. I could get no orders from him; and the ADMS divisions were pressing me for stores and equipment from my Advanced Depots Medical Stores which I felt they were not entitled to, and over which I turned out to be right later. 'Let them have them,' was all I got out from the General. Egypt kept asking for information, which I tried to give them; [...].
>
> I did all I could meanwhile to shield the DMS because I liked him very much. He was a sound administrator. [...] I sensed that there was trouble brewing at GHQ. [...] Two days later the blow fell. The DMS was superseded, and the DDMS of the 20th Corps, Colonel Richard Luce, appointed in his place.[16]

It was General Allenby himself who decided to relieve General Swan of his command. The C-in-C had known him from the Western Front, trusted him, and relied on him. It was Allenby who had brought him from the VII Corps of the 3rd Army in France to be DMS of the EEF in Palestine. Yet, he did not hesitate to take the difficult decision concerning Surgeon General Swan when he thought that the fate of the offensive's medical organization might be at stake.

With hindsight, one cannot refrain from the thought that General Swan was a victim of Post Traumatic Stress Disorder (PTSD) – inability to function after a traumatic event. This psychiatric entity was known at the time as 'shell shock' and this mainly on the Western Front, where it was very slowly recognized as a real medical problem. General Swan, like many others, did not have any opportunity to undergo diagnosis or treatment in Palestine at that time due to the lack of proper professional attitude and knowledge. He died not too long after being relieved of his post.[17]

During the night of 16 September, the Arab army, led by Sheikh Feisal and Lt-Col. Lawrence, attacked the Hejaz railway in three different sites around Der'a. This attack served the cause of deception by diverting full attention to the area east of the Jordan. Chaytor's Force actively continued its diversionary demonstrations in the Jordan Valley. During the coming days, British airplanes bombed several targets around Amman and Der'a in addition to other enemy targets, including Nablus. During the night of 18 September the XX Corps attacked in the Judean hills, also serving the diversion. Several formations, including the 60th Division, moved to their attack positions during the night, escaping notice by the enemy.

At 0445 on 19 September, after a heavy artillery barrage that lasted for fifteen minutes, the XXI corps attacked according to plan. It was supported by fire from two Royal Navy monitors, the 'Druid' and the 'Forester,' aimed at the line of Nahr el Falik. Resistance was encountered mainly in the eastern sector, where the 54th Division and the French detachment were fighting. By 0730 the enemy's front line had been breached and the hidden cavalry divisions began to advance through the lines; by 1030 the battle in the plain was over and the entire XXI Corps turned eastward as planned. All the objectives were taken as expected; the 60th Division, which had marched altogether seventeen miles, reached Tul Karm and captured it by evening. The 5th Australian Light Horse Brigade, which had begun the fighting with the 60th Division, left it after the enemy line had been breached, rode into the mountains and reached the Mesudie Junction where it cut off the enemy's possible retreat route.

By mid-day the mounted forces crossed Nahr Iskanderune and reached Liktera. The 5th Cavalry Division sent a reconnoitring force into the Abu Shushe route while the 4th Cavalry Division sent a detachment to Wadi Ara in the direction of the Musmus pass. The VIII Turkish army ceased to exist as a military organization as most of its troops were either taken prisoner or were on the run.

The number of casualties was much less than expected.[18] Until the complete destruction of the VIII and VII Turkish armies, the EEF suffered about 5,000 casualties. The XXI Corps, which was by far the largest one and had carried the main assault, sustained 3,378 casualties, only 446 of them killed; 2,619 were wounded and 313 missing in action.[19] The XX Corps suffered 1,505 casualties during the same period of time: 225 dead, 1,262 wounded, and 18 missing. The number of casualties in the Desert Mounted Corps and Chaytor's Force was minimal.

The medical services operated methodically and efficiently, exactly according to plan. The DDMSs and the ADMSs cooperated with one another, maintaining enough flexibility to change medical units' missions when needed. Full cooperation was also attained from the staff officers at all levels. Cooperation with the Deputy Adjutant-General EEF and the Deputy Quarter-Master General EEF was excellent. As the actual number of casualties was much lower than estimated and there were enough medical units which could cooperate in their work, no medical facility was overwhelmed by a sudden unexpected wave of a huge number of casualties.

Immediately after the enemy front line was breached and captured, a water pipeline some 7,000 yards long, with an output of 17,500 water gallons per hour, was laid by the XXI Corps RE unit from Farkhie to Jiljulie in eight-and-a-half hours.[20]

Some of the field ambulances had difficulty in keeping pace with the mounted divisions due to the nature of the terrain and bad roads. One field ambulance returned through the lines and eventually made its way to Tul Karm. The immobile sections of the field ambulances opened dressing stations along their routes, and then found that they could move forward much faster without their heavy equipment. They managed to notify the ADMS L-of-C, hoping he would know what to do. Though it seems the ADMS did not like the situation too much, he simply had no choice, or, in his own words:

> Another trouble also now overtook us. The troops were moving so quickly onwards, and the Field Ambulances with them, that it was found the latter could not keep up without shedding part of their equipment. So all day, and each day for several days, we of the L-of-C were getting messages by dispatch rider like this: 'Have had to abandon part of equipment at El Tirah (or Tul-Keram or Musmus further and further away each time). Please collect.' Just that: 'Please collect.' No suggestion of how the L-of-C, which possesses no wheeled transport of its own, could collect.
>
> Now a Field Ambulance in those days was worth about £20,000, and we did not want valuable equipment to be looted by wandering Bedouin; so with Major Munro I crossed the broken Turkish front to have a look round, and see if we could arrange for empty returning ration lorries to pick up our equipment.[21]

During the night of 19 September the XX Corps attacked according to plan. Though both divisions faced resistance, they managed to overcome it and advance to the Nablus road, capturing it during the afternoon of the 20th. The Royal Flying Corps attacked retreating Turkish convoys anywhere they were spotted. The 3rd and 7th Divisions of the XXI Corps continued to advance during that day, converging towards Mesudie Junction where they joined up with the 5th Australian Light Horse Brigade.

Early on 20 September the cavalry brigades reached the Esdraelon Valley, not far from the site of the ancient city of Megiddo, the biblical Armageddon. The 5th Division remained at El Affule and sent the 13th Brigade to raid General Liman von Sanders' GHQ at Nazareth. The raiding force entered Nazareth so quickly that the Turkish GHQ was taken by complete surprise and General von Sanders himself barely escaped. The 4th Cavalry Division continued to Beisan which was captured at 1630 after a ride of 85 miles in 34 hours. The 19th Lancers Regiment of the same division continued northward and during the night seized the important bridge across the Jordan at El Majamie. The 4th Light Horse Brigade of the Australian Mounted Division, which advanced next to the 4th Cavalry Division, reached Jenin by the evening. There, 'a fully equipped German hospital staffed by trained army nurses, 300 enemy patients were found.'[22] The hospital was still fully operating.

Thus, by the end of that day most possible routes for Turkish retreat were blocked by mounted units. British airplanes continued to raid the retreating Turkish units everywhere, contributing much to their insecurity and despair. About 25,000 prisoners were captured during the first day of the offensive.

During 21 September the XXI Corps' infantry divisions accomplished their objectives and were concentrating and reorganizing at various locations. The XX Corps' divisions were still fighting their way to Nablus which was captured by the end of the day. When the medical units entered Nablus they found more than four hundred Turkish sick and wounded soldiers at the English hospital in the town. Though they were well treated, the hospital teams were exhausted. A medical unit composed of No. 74 CCS with mobile bacteriologic laboratory and a section of the 171 Combined Field Ambulance immediately took charge of the hospital and continued the medical work there.[23]

Units of the XX Corps reached the Jordan Valley and blocked the roads leading from eastwards from Nablus. During this day the 13th Brigade of the 5th Cavalry Division captured Nazareth. Most of the mounted units were engaged in rounding up prisoners of war. By the end of 21 September, the victory over the Turkish armies west of the Jordan was complete and the infantry divisions had accomplished their very important role in the offensive. General Allenby was so confident of success that he wrote on that very same day to his wife: 'I think the Turkish Army is practically destroyed.'[24]

Chaytor's Force maintained active defence and was engaged in minor encounters with the enemy along the Jordan Valley front. On 21 September it advanced to the Damiye Bridge, establishing connection with XX Corps units west of the Jordan and with cavalry units east of Jenin. On 22 September, it continued to press hard northwards and by evening the New Zealand Mounted Brigade captured the Damiye Bridge. Later during the night Chaytor's Force began to climb eastwards along the familiar routes to Es Salt.

The 5th Cavalry Division was concentrated at this time in Nazareth, preparing to attack Haifa and Acre. A detachment of armoured cars which had approached Haifa on the main road faced heavy fire and was forced to fall back. The 15th Brigade failed to take Haifa in the first attempt. A coordinated assault on Haifa, consisting of a frontal attack together with one from the rear on the garrison's artillery, located on Mount Carmel, brought about the capture of Haifa. On 23 September, in the afternoon, Chaytor's Force reached Es Salt and the 13th Brigade of the 5th Cavalry Division captured Acre without any resistance.

During the night of 24 September the 4th Australian Light Horse Brigade took Samakh after a difficult hand-to-hand battle with the local German garrison. The force then moved on to Tiberias, arriving there when an outbreak of cholera occurred among the residents of this town. The source of the outbreak was the contaminated drinking water of the Lake of Galilee. The forces could not avoid the passing through Tiberias, as it was located on the only available road to Damascus. However, they were ordered not to have any contact with the local population. As a result, only one soldier fell sick with cholera. The town's population was treated efficiently by a group of American Jewish volunteer doctors and nurses who established medical services in the town at that time.[25]

In all these operations there were very few casualties and the medical units continued to be engaged mainly in treating sick and wounded Turkish prisoners. The worst situation was in Nazareth. Though there were several hospitals in the town, they were all overcrowded and disorganized. Only on 27 September, when the DADMS of the Desert Mounted Corps came to Nazareth, was a solution found. He brought with him two Divisional Receiving Stations which moved into the hospitals and took charge of their work.

On 25 September Chaytor's Force captured Amman and the railway north of Amman. In the town itself, the staffs of two Turkish hospitals were doing their best, treating about 480 sick and wounded patients. Within twenty-four hours the number of sick at the hospitals rose to more than 1,000. They were eventually evacuated by motor lorries to Jerusalem with the Turkish medical staff. A Dressing Station was simultaneously opened at the ruins of Amman's Roman amphitheatre.

All this time General Chaytor was looking forward to the inevitable encounter with the Turkish Army II Corps that was retreating from Hejaz and Ma'an. This corps, part of the IV Turkish Army, was ordered to retreat northwards, its route to Damascus leading through the Amman area. It was retreating on foot, for the railroad was already out of use. Aware of the fact that the only water source available for the retreating Turkish force was at Wadi el Hammam, the 1st Australian Light Horse Brigade was sent to capture it. The 2nd Light Horse Brigade moved southward waiting for the II Corps' arrival. It was located by airplane reconnaissance on the 27th, and following negotiations with commanding officers of the Light Horse who explained to the Turkish commanders their desperate situation, the entire Turkish force of about 4,500 men surrendered on 29 September. About 500 men of this force were so ill that they had to be evacuated to Jerusalem; the rest were taken to Amman.[26] With the surrender of the Turkish II Corps, the mission of Chaytor's Force had been very successfully accomplished. Since 19 September it had taken captive more than 10,000 prisoners and captured Amman. During that time it had sustained only 139 casualties.

Meanwhile, the C-in-C was planning the next phase of the campaign. Since he believed that the objectives of the Battle of Megiddo had not been achieved as long as the Turkish IV Army continued to exist, the campaign must continue. On 22 September General Allenby met General Chauvel at the Desert Mounted Corps Advanced HQ at Lajjun. It was the first time that Allenby revealed to another party his plans for the future campaign. Though this was still before the capture of Acre, Haifa, Samakh, and Tiberias, the C-in-C was quite confident about the progress of the immediate operations and anxious to continue the momentum.

General Allenby's plan called for destruction of the retreating IV Army on its way to Damascus. This could be achieved by cavalry forces in cooperation with the Arab army. Thus, two cavalry divisions, the Australian Mounted Division and the 5th Cavalry Division, were to cross the Jordan north of the Lake of Galilee and advance toward Damascus through El Quneitra. The 4th Cavalry Division would cross the Jordan south of the Lake of Galilee and proceed eastwards in the direction of Der'a. It would establish contact with the Arab army near Der'a, then advance northwards in the direction of Damascus. All Desert Mounted Corps units were instructed to take up defensive positions on the high ground commanding Damascus and to encircle it, but not to enter the city. For political reasons, Damascus itself would be taken by the Arab army, though with the assistance of EEF cavalry units.[27] An official order for the advance on Damascus was issued by the EEF General Staff on 26 September.[28] It also ordered the XXI Corps to be ready to advance with one of its divisions from Haifa to Beirut.

The unsolved problem raised by this plan was the issue of supplies: since the railroads in the area were not functioning and the cavalry was expected to advance at a fast pace, no practical feasible way of supplying the force was found. It was decided that the troops would carry two days' supplies for themselves and a one-day supply for the horses. A lorry supply convoy would follow the force to El Quneitra. This, however, would not solve the supply problems of the 4th Cavalry Division which was directed 'to requisite supplies on its march.'[29]

Medical evacuation during the planned operations did not seem to be a crucial problem, as only few casualties were expected and all the brigades were to be followed by their field ambulances. Despite this optimistic assessment, it was planned that the lorries returning from El Quneitra would bring with them casualties from the medical stations of the brigades of the Australian Mounted and the 5th Divisions. They were expected to evacuate them to the hospital in Nazareth or to the reinforced Combined Field Ambulance which arrived at Samakh at that time.

Famous for describing events in understatement, on 26 September General Allenby's order of the day to the EEF troops proclaimed: 'Such a complete victory has seldom been known in all the history of war.'[30]

On 27 September the Australian Mounted Division, the 5th Cavalry Division, and the HQ of the Desert Mounted Corps began their advance northwards. They found that the Jisr Benat el Yakub – the main bridge over the Jordan – had been partially demolished by retreating Turkish forces. The brigades then began to cross the river under fire, successfully doing so in several fords, and drove the enemy out of its positions. There were only few casualties during the crossing, inflicted by one of the enemy's last air attacks. By dusk on 28 September the Desert Mounted Corps reached El Quneitra and in the evening of the 29th it was fighting its way through the Sa'sa area, south of Damascus.

The 4th Cavalry Division crossed the Jordan south of the Lake of Galilee to intercept the retreating IV Turkish Army. By that time, the IV Army troops, deprived of sleep, thirsty and hungry, were concentrated in the area of Der'a–Muzeirib, seventy-five miles south of Damascus. During the night of 27 September the Arab troops achieved a real military success when they captured Der'a. When the 4th Cavalry Division entered Der'a the next day, they could only watch in horror the outcome of that victory:

> A grim spectacle was needed to shock the troops of the cavalry division which for ten days had been harrying the retreat of a routed army; but the sight of Der'a station and its encampments

> that met the 10th Cavalry Brigade as it rode in that morning was ghastly beyond aught that any man there had yet witnessed. Everywhere there were dead Turks, but they were the fortunate; for the wounded lay scattered about, despoiled and in agony, amid a litter of packages, half looted, half burnt, of torn documents, and smashed machinery. A hospital train stood in the station; the driver and fireman were still in their cab, still alive, but mortally wounded; the sick and wounded in the train have been stripped of every rag of clothing.

'In the whole course of this war,' wrote Major General Barrow, OC 4th Cavalry Division, 'in France and in Palestine, I have never seen such a sight of dreadful misery.' After establishing contact with the Arab army and arranging the details of cooperation during the advance on Damascus, the 4th Division began to move north, but not before 'the 10th Brigade piqueted the station, collected and dressed the Turkish wounded, and buried the dead.'[31]

At midnight of 30 September, the Desert Mounted Corps troops reined in their horses at the gates of Damascus.

9

THE LAST PHASE: THE RIDERS AND THE APOCALYPSE

'From a medical point of view, the most important problem of this Campaign – as of all previous campaigns in this country – has been that of malaria.'

A Brief Record of the Advance of the Egyptian Expeditionary Force under the Command of General Sir Edmund H.H. Allenby, July 1917 to October 1918, 2d ed. (London: HMSO, 1919), 105.

'The report of the Committee of Enquiry regarding the prevalence of Pellagra among Turkish prisoners of war will stand for years to come as a record of one of the best and most scientific inquiries ever accomplished by a nation at war.'

'Medicine in the War – Second Notice,' *British Medical Journal* (1922) part II: 761–62.

On 1 October 1918 Arab army troops entered Damascus as conquerors. Units of the Desert Mounted Corps, which had been encircling Damascus since the previous night, were allowed to enter the city after them. According to prior political agreements, the Arabs were expected to administrate the captured city and run its municipal services. T.E. Lawrence described the situation he encountered: 'The streets were full of the debris of the broken army, derelict carts and cars, baggage, material, corpses. Typhus, dysentery and pellagra were rife among the Turks, and sufferers had died in every shadow along the line of march.'[1] In very short time all concerned realized that the task was too demanding for the Arab force, which lacked any administrative infrastructure and without which no practical problem could be solved.

The main problem facing the new rulers of Damascus was prisoners of war. About 20,000 Turks were taken captive in the Damascus area. Thousands of them were sick and wounded soldiers who had been abandoned by their retreating units in various hospitals around the city. As the hospitals were understaffed and lacked food and medical provisions, many of these patients were in terrible condition.[2]

Major W. Evans, the DADMS of the Australian Mounted Division and one of the first medical personnel to enter the military hospital at the Hamidie Barracks, commented: 'Condition of 600–700 patients in this hospital was found on inspection to be indescribably hideous and inhuman. Deserted by all save a handful of Turkish Medical personnel, starved for three days, and suffocated by the stench of their own offal and the unburied dead, the plight of these wretches was more than miserable.'[3] There were five other hospitals in the city, in some of which the patients were in an even worse condition.

The most crowded hospital was at the Beramkie Barracks, where 900 wounded and sick Turkish soldiers were lying under horrible conditions in two buildings. The hospital staff consisted of seven Syrian doctors who worked continuously without any help. There was neither food nor medical stores. Another medical facility was the Merkaz Hospital, where 650 patients were hospitalized. Though this was the only fully staffed hospital, it lacked administrative services and as a result the patients suffered from lack of food and medical comforts. Three hospitals were located in the Bab Tuma area. One was the English Hospital, fully occupied by 130 patients, whose medical personnel had fled. Professional activity, as well as all other work, was performed by three British nurses who had been brought there by the retreating Turks from a hospital in Nazareth.[4] There were 107 patients at the French Hospital who were treated by only one doctor. At the German Hospital there were 350 patients, most of them Germans. Sixteen of the patients were captured Australian soldiers. They were all treated by one very dedicated German medical officer, himself sick, who was assisted by local untrained staff. Four hundred slightly wounded soldiers were hospitalized in several houses in the vicinity of the hospitals. They were unattended and had no food or medical comforts. More than 2,000 sick and wounded Turkish troops were in the Kadem Hospital, in the southern sector of the city, many of them in a desperate state of health. They were attended by four Turkish medical officers and a few orderlies, who had neither medical equipment nor any supplies.

Altogether, when Damascus fell to the British and Arab forces there were more than three thousand hospitalized Turkish soldiers who were receiving inadequate treatment.[5]

When General Chauvel heard from his medical officers about conditions at the various hospitals in the city, and being aware of the incompetent Arab administration, he decided that treatment of prisoners of war was the responsibility of the Desert Mounted Corps. After four days of Arab army administration, Desert Mounted Corps troops took control of the hospitals. Chauvel issued an order appointing his DDMS, Colonel Downes, as the senior Medical Officer of the city, responsible for all aspects of health and medicine there. Major W. Evans, the DADMS of the Australian Mounted Division, was appointed by Colonel Downes to supervise the hospitals. As expected, the Arab authorities considered this an act of interference with their administration of the city, and refused to accept it. They suggested that Captain Ramsey, RAMC, a Medical Officer who served with the Arab army, would be responsible for the hospitals in the city.[6] After negotiations, a compromise was reached: Colonel Downes remained the senior Medical Officer in Damascus, while Captain Ramsey would supervise the hospitals but report to Colonel Downes. Major Evans continued to work with Colonel Downes at the hospitals without formal appointment.[7]

The team immediately got to work. Under Major Evans' orders healthy prisoners of war from nearby prison camps were sent to clean the Beramkie Hospital and bury the dead. All other hospitals were cleaned and organized for Turkish casualties. Turkish Medical Officers and medical orderlies who were found among the many prisoners of war were also sent to work in the hospitals. Local people too were recruited for assistance. In order to concentrate all efforts and maximize efficiency, all the 1,137 patients in the Kadem Hospital were transferred to Merkaz and Beramkie Hospitals. A non-combatant NCO was appointed quartermaster to every hospital. Under the efforts directed by Colonel Downes, the death rate among the hospitalized Turkish patients decreased from seventy per day on 3 October to fifteen per day a week later. The French and English Hospitals at Bab Tuma were prepared to admit future sick troops from the Desert Mounted Corps brigades.

During the first few days after the fall of Damascus only the mobile sections of the field ambulances could reach the city, and there was no L-of-C at all.[8] The outcome was that a severe shortage in medical supplies was developing very quickly. Medical stores were found in various locations in the city itself; some of them were purchased and others, which were found to be stolen from hospitals, were confiscated. Urgent medical supplies were brought to Damascus by airplanes from Palestine. Only on 5 October did supplies arrive from Samakh through the Benat Yakub Bridge. On 12 October an Advanced Operating Unit arrived in Damascus and took charge of the French Hospital, while a section of the 3rd Australian Light Horse Field Ambulance took over the English Mission Hospital.

There were also severe difficulties in evacuating patients from Damascus to hospitals in the rear, there being only one feasible route leaving the city towards the southwest and leading to Samakh. This road was so difficult to travel that all seriously ill EEF personnel and all sick Turks were retained in Damascus, with only slightly ill EEF soldiers being sent by motor lorries to Samakh. However, the journey had to be divided into stages. The first, a distance of forty-two miles, was to El Quneitra, where a mobile section of the 4th Light Horse Field Ambulance took over the patients for the night. The second stage was to Rosh-Pina, where a Receiving Station of the 4th Cavalry Division was located. Finally, the patients were evacuated another fifty miles to No. 33 Combined Clearing Hospital in Haifa. The harbour in Haifa had been working at full capacity since 27 September, enabling the evacuation of patients from Haifa to Egypt by hospital ships.[9]

There was an extreme shortage of vehicles for medical evacuation during the first days after the occupation of Damascus. Priority at that time was given to evacuation from the city of as many prisoners of war as possible, in order to diminish the need for food. Eventually it was decided that returning supply lorries would evacuate prisoners of war, while returning ammunition lorries would be committed to medical evacuation.[10] During the first days of October no large-scale military operations were undertaken. As a result, there were only very few battle casualties, allowing the medical units at all levels to reorganize and be able to deal with the cardinal problem of that time: the health problems of the Turkish prisoners of war.

While all this was happening in Damascus, the 7th Infantry Division of the XXI Corps made its way from Haifa to Beirut. On 4 October it reached the town of Tyre, where it was supplied from the sea for three more days.

It was supplied again from the sea when it reached Sidon on 6 October. By the evening of 8 October the force reached Beirut. Throughout its advance the 7th Division had not faced any resistance.

On 5 October the Desert Mounted Corps, less the Australian Mounted Division, resumed its advance. That division was retained in the Damascus area to maintain order there. It established a Division Collecting Station for slight cases in a building at El Mezze. The 4th and the 5th Cavalry Divisions of the Desert Mounted Corps moved towards Mu'allaqa and Rayak. When they faced no resistance at Rayak, one of the main railway junctions in Syria, the divisions began advancing in the direction of Ba'albek. On its way, the 4th Division established a hospital at Buldan, some twenty miles northwest of Damascus, while the 5th Division established a hospital at Mu'allaqa. Three days later the L-of -C was extended to include Damascus, Mu'allaqa, and Beirut. No. 66 CCS arrived in Damascus and established itself at the Baramkie Barracks Hospital. No. 32 Combined Clearing Hospital from Jerusalem and No.15 Combined Clearing Hospital from Rantie arrived at Beirut.

Their arrival at Beirut facilitated the process of medical evacuation from Damascus and from the mounted brigades advancing northwards. There was no more need for evacuation to hospitals in Palestine through Samakh. Patients from Damascus could be evacuated to Beirut through Mu'allaqa and from Beirut by hospital ships directly to hospitals in Egypt, mainly to Port Said. From 19 October on, supplies were landed at Beirut harbour from where they were transported through Mu'allaqa to Damascus and later to Ba'albek for the 4th and 5th Cavalry Divisions.

On 9 October General Allenby ordered the Desert Mounted Corps to advance on Homs. It seemed that the Turkish army, or what remained of it, had already retired northwards in order to establish a defence line in the vicinity of Aleppo. It was assumed that no resistance was expected and that the pace of advance would depend only on supplies. Allenby accepted Sheikh Feisal's offer that an Arab mounted unit of 1,500 cavalrymen and camel-mounted troops would advance with the Desert Mounted Corps to secure its right flank and operate against Turkish communications between Homs and Aleppo. The Desert Mounted Corps divisions reached Ba'albek on 10 October and found it deserted, as expected. However, at Ba'albek it was realized that the 4th Division could not continue its advance due to the mounting number of sick soldiers.

Malaria began to affect all the Desert Mounted Corps brigades, but it affected mainly the 4th Cavalry Division already as it made its way to Damascus. As predicted, about ten days after the division had camped in Beisan, 'one of the most unhealthiest places in Palestine,'[11] and a week after both the 5th Cavalry and the Australian Mounted Divisions spent a night near the Benat Yakub Bridge, the troops began to suffer from high fever and rigors, typical symptoms of malaria. The disease spread much more quickly when the corps reached Damascus – within a few days more than half the troops were sick with malaria of the malignant type. While during the week previous to the capture of Damascus the rate of hospital admissions was 2.85 percent of the force, the following week it became 5.51 percent. 'Nearly four times as many men of the Corps died in Damascus as had been killed between the beginning of the offensive and the capture of Damascus.'[12] At Ba'albek the 4th Cavalry Division became immobilized as its losses through malignant malaria were so high 'that not enough men were left to attend to the horse-lines, and its further employment became impossible.'[13] One of the 4th Cavalry Division troops wrote his family:

> I am afraid that I must now relate the saddest period of my war experiences – as it saw the end of my active service, and very nearly the end of my life. On the way between Damascus and Ba'albek, we contracted it [malaria] in the Jordan Valley. There was no quinine and no medical aid had managed to keep up with us. Several of my friends died.[14]

It was suggested that the Australian Mounted Division, which was stationed around Damascus at that time and had sustained less than one hundred casualties since the beginning of the offensive, would replace the 4th Division. However, it could not join the 5th Cavalry Division according to the timetable dictated by the C-in-C. Thus, the 5th Division, which had spent but one night at the Jordan Valley and the number of its sick was the lowest, remained the only cavalry force capable of advancing northwards. It was ready to continue the advance supported only by Arab army cavalrymen. The 5th Division reached Homs on 16 October and found that the Turkish forces had deserted it. The division's supplies problem was solved quite easily by requisitioning food and forage from local inhabitants along the route of advance. The advancing force rested at Homs for three days awaiting new orders.

During that time the 7th Infantry Division advanced along the coast from Beirut and took Tripoli without any resistance on 18 October. It was replaced in Beirut three days later by the 54th Division of the XXI Corps. The capture of Tripoli again shortened to a great degree the routes of supply and of medical evacuation from Syria, as Tripoli harbour could be used for these purposes. In a few days No. 74 CCS was established in Tripoli.

The main problem, however, remained the health of the forces in the Damascus area. While many soldiers took ill with malignant malaria, a new scourge was on its way. The pandemic of influenza named 'The Spanish Flue,' which had already affected the armies on the Western Front, arrived in Damascus on 6 October 1918. When Spanish Flue affected the German troops fighting on the Western Front during the spring of 1918, this epidemic was blamed by some of the senior German commanders as one of the reasons for the failure of the large German Spring Offensive. This claim ignored the fact that both the British and the French troops facing them suffered from the epidemic as well.[15] The Spanish Flue of 1918–19 was the most devastating pandemic of the twentieth century. It killed over twenty million people around the world – many more than died in combat during the entire Great War. It was a specific virulent form of influenza which, contrary to other forms of this disease, affected mainly young healthy people. Its main clinical manifestations were high fever and severe infection with oedema of the respiratory tract. In many cases the influenza was complicated by pneumonia which led to death in some of them.[16]

In the medical context of Damascus, the appearance of the Spanish Flue precisely when many British troops and Turkish prisoners of war were being treated for malaria posed a serious problem for the medical services. Though there was no specific treatment for the flue, which was treated symptomatically, there might always be patients who suffered from both diseases and urgently needed intravenous quinine therapy. Thus, the diagnosis of malaria had to be made immediately. On the other hand, accurate diagnosis was necessary so as not to waste quinine when it was not needed. There was always a shortage of quinine which was supplied to the troops in inadequate quantities.[17]

The medical situation in Damascus was again on the verge of a catastrophe: since the capture of the city and the initial organization of the local hospitals, 8,250 new cases of sick Turkish prisoners of war, suffering either from malaria or from Spanish Flue, had been admitted to the hospitals already filled to capacity. In addition, thousands of EEF soldiers suffering from the same diseases were pouring into the various medical installations: 1,246 soldiers of the Desert Mounted Corps were admitted to hospitals in Damascus during the week ending 5 October. During the next week, until 12 October, 3,109 additional troops were admitted to the various medical installations.[18] This was one of the finest hours of the medical service. Teams consisting of medical officers and orderlies, themselves taken ill, did not leave their patients for a moment, doing anything they could for them. The medical teams took care of food and drinking water, as well as caring for the patients' hygiene and welfare. However, they were mainly engaged in alleviating the symptoms of Spanish Flue and giving intravenous injections of quinine, in order to rescue the patients from the deadly malignant malaria. Many of these soldiers were evacuated from the hospitals in Damascus to one of the harbours and thence to a hospital in Egypt where they had better prospects of recovering. Though the medical services everywhere did the best they could, the toll was high. During October and November 1918, 479 soldiers died of the diseases they had contracted, more than four times the number of Desert Mounted Corps soldiers who were killed on the battlefield since the offensive had commenced.[19]

The simultaneous outbreak of two severe diseases at Damascus was quite an unusual phenomenon which called for some unusual solutions to cope with it. During that extreme situation the humanistic approach of several Australian officers was noted. These officers, who did not belong to the medical services, cared for the prisoners of war in their camps, supported them and did everything they could for their welfare. No doubt, this attitude was inspired by General Chauvel's own approach that was clearly evident after the capture of Damascus. Malaria and Spanish Flue affected EEF units and Turkish prisoners everywhere. The medical teams, who were not immune to the diseases, were as sick as the rest of the troops, yet they had to carry on and care for their patients until they were relieved by other medical teams.

Diseases, mainly malaria, affected units not only in the Damascus area. Dr Redcliffe N. Salaman, the Medical Officer of the 39th Royal Fusiliers, which was a part of Chaytor's Force, was especially bitter:

> The medical side of the campaign, as you will have guessed, has fairly broken down, the failure being entirely due to lack of knowledge and foresight on the part of the senior administrative medical officers. Preparations had been made on a considerable

> scale for the wounded; but when it appeared that there were but few, the extra beds were packed up and sent to ordnance; at the same time, evacuation of the hospitals had been left till too late and, crowning mistake of all, they had forgotten that the autumn was the season for malaria and that the disease took ten days to incubate. The consequence was that just when the old men were preening their feathers and thinking of the decorations that would be theirs, and how wonderfully their poorly devised schemes had coped with the casualties, out broke the most tremendous epidemic of malaria.
>
> The cases poured in from everywhere, but nowhere heavier than on our side; hospital transport between Salt and Jerusalem utterly failed – the R.A.S.C. saved the situation. At every halt I had to fight to get my men evacuated; between halts many had just dropped out on the side of the road and been picked up – by a passing lorry. To add to one's difficulties the returning lorries from Amman and Es Salt were often packed with sick prisoners, and, in that way, very often they had precedence of our own sick. When we got to this camp in Jerusalem I got one of the Hadassa medical men to examine blood films for me, and, as I had expected, the great majority of our sick were malaria cases and about 70 per cent of them malignant.[20]

The fact was that soldiers of Chaytor's Force began to suffer from malaria several days after the Force advanced into the previously Turkish-occupied area in the Jordan Valley.

However, there were other sides to this problem as well. One of them was recorded by the ADMS L-of-C:

> One curious episode happening at that time was the complete disappearance of a cavalry squadron. It got lost somewhere on the way to Damascus; and it was the job of the L. of C. to find it. We were searching rather casually when one of our staff, Lieutenant-Colonel McLeod, riding along the ridge over Mount Carmel, spotted what looked like horse lines in the plain below, and thought he'd like to investigate. When he went down he

> saw at once it was the lost squadron, but then to his surprise he found a German N.C.O. in charge. The N.C.O. explained that he and the other Germans were prisoners of war who had been captured by the squadron, that all the British were down with influenza, and that he and his comrades were looking after them. The Germans, he said, had not attempted to escape. They had no desire to do so and have their throats cut by the Arabs. So they remained.[21]

During October and November 1918 Chaytor's Force, which had commenced the operation with 13,000 men, lost 8,352 of them to malaria (and maybe also to the Spanish Flue). Many of the sick soldiers died of the disease. Compare this figure with only 139 casualties that it had suffered since the beginning of the September advance.[22] It is not difficult to understand why the Medical Officer was infuriated, especially when 'the most unfortunate would appear to have been the 1st and 2nd Light Horse Brigades, the only troops in the theatre engaged from the day when Murray's Forces first advanced across the Suez Canal.'[23]

As if all these health and medical problems were not enough, the medical services had to face a new and previously unknown one. Already at the beginning of October 1918, after the capture of Damascus, an outbreak of a disease identified as Pellagra affected many of the Turkish prisoners of war who were kept in special camps. That disease was soon diagnosed in 9,257 out of 105,668 Turkish prisoners. There were probably many more cases whose clinical manifestations were milder and thus went unnoticed and undiagnosed.

Pellagra was a medical condition unknown to most European physicians. Though the disease had been first described in Europe, during the eighteenth century, it was quite rare there. Only few of the physicians working at the time in Egypt were familiar with it.[24] The clinical manifestations of Pellagra were severe diarrhoea and severe skin lesions accompanied by oedema, mainly of the limbs. It could also affect the central nervous system, causing neurological disturbances and dementia. In many cases the disease was fatal. While it was easy to diagnose Pellagra, due to its typical combination of clinical manifestations, its etiology remained obscure at the time. Furthermore, there was no consensus among physicians concerning its treatment.

No wonder, then, that the EEF medical services became very concerned

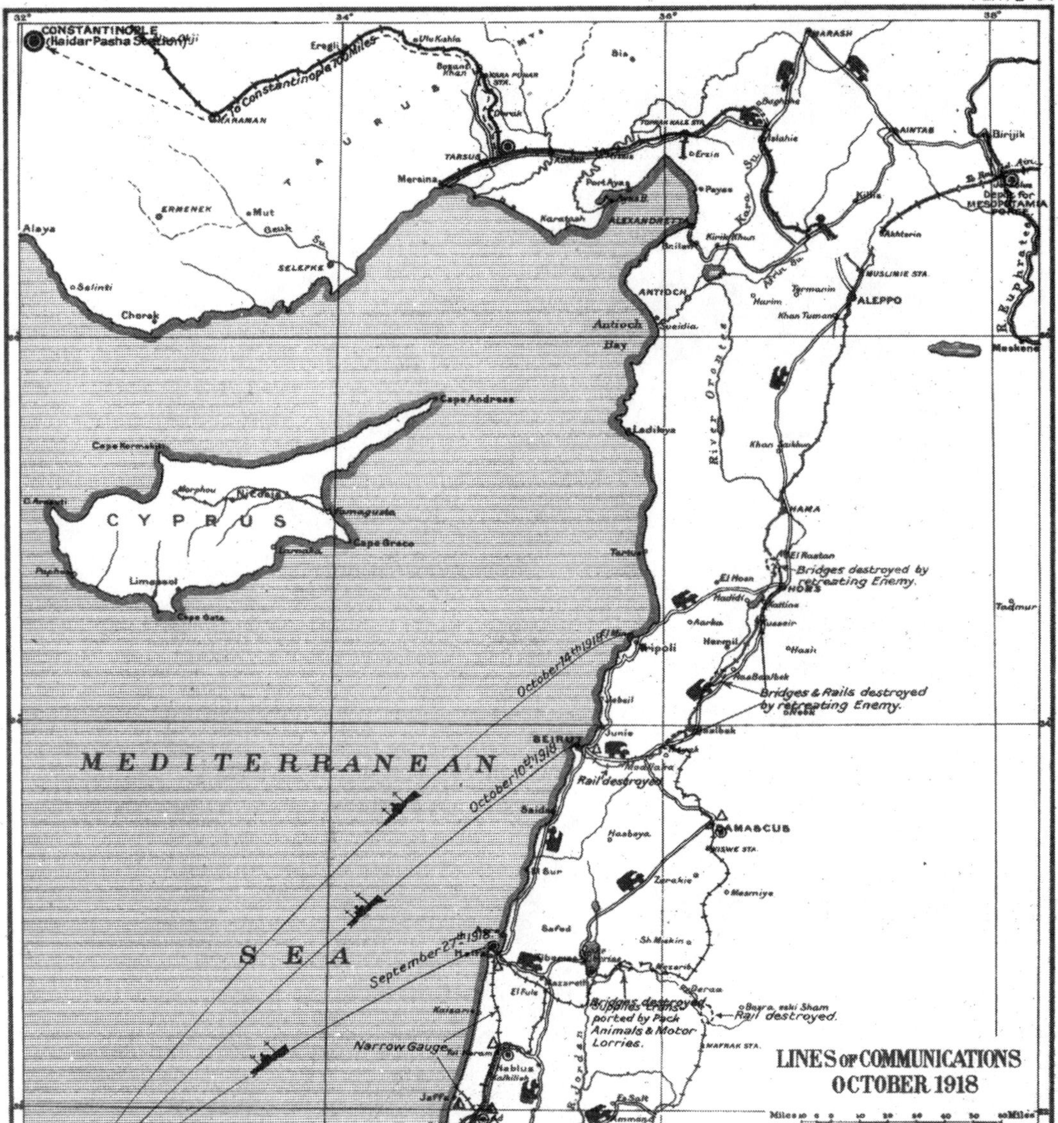

Reproduced by the Survey of Egypt Dec 1918 (6453)

Reprinted in England 1919.

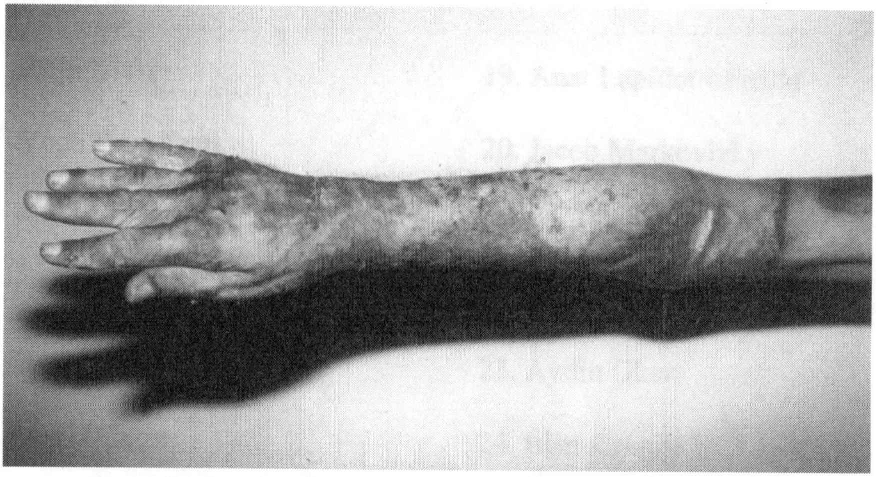

A Turkish POW suffering from Pellagra

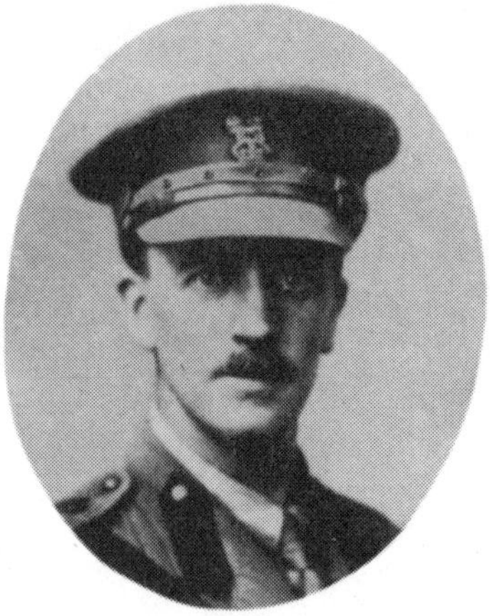

Col Rupert M. Downes

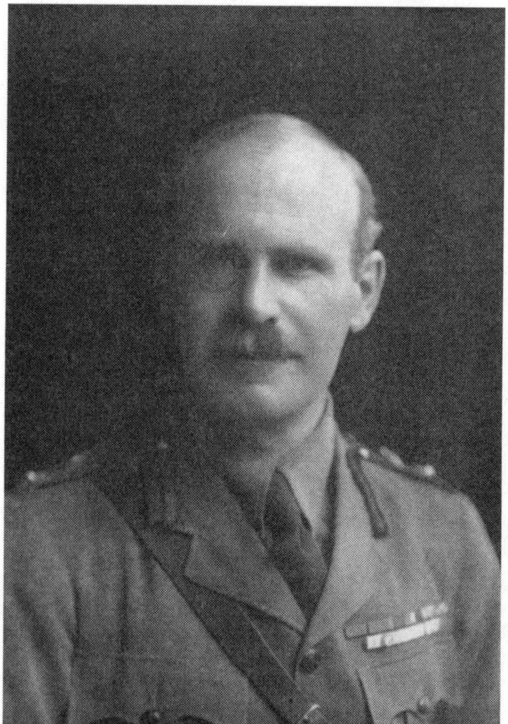

Lt Col J Johnston Abraham

when the disease, so prevalent among the Turkish prisoners, was diagnosed by the experts as Pellagra. The main concern of the DMS was quite simple: a disease whose etiology was unknown might be contagious and affect the EEF troops as well.

It was General Allenby who promptly responded to the news of the Pellagra outbreak among the Turkish prisoners. He decided to inquire into the nature of this disease for three reasons, the first being his assumption that investigating the outbreak of Pellagra in the military setting created an opportunity which might not recur of ascertaining the true nature of Pellagra. The C-in-C also thought that everything should be done to prevent the spread of this disease from the Turkish prisoners to British troops and that the first step should be to understand its causes and nature. The third reason was Allenby's judgement that a future serious political attack at home was inevitable, in view of the devastation caused among the prisoners of war.[25] General Allenby wrote to the CIGS, General Wilson:

> Sickness is troubling us. I had the mosquitos well in hand; and soon the Jordan valley had become almost a summer health resort. Now I'm in Turkish territory, and malignant malaria is laying a lot of people by the heels. I've a good acting DMS now; one Luce; and he is doing all he can, but his beds are all full. I want to send some thousands of sick to Malta; but Salonika appears to have filled up most of the beds there. My Turkish prisoners are improving in health, to some extent, and their death-rate is diminishing. Thousands are still in Damascus, awaiting removal to Egypt, but transport is not sufficient.[26]

Allenby's attitude – that the nature of the disease should be investigated while the war was still being waged – was very unusual. However, it was typical of Allenby, who had always been interested in the health problems among his troops. He immediately directed the DMS EEF, Surgeon General Luce, to investigate the problem of Pellagra.

On 6 October the DMS appointed Col. F.G. Boyd, one of the senior consulting physicians to the EEF, and Lt-Col. P.S. Lelean, an authority on sanitation and epidemiology, as members of the enquiry committee. The committee's terms of reference were in accord with General Allenby's outlook: they were quite broad, covering practically all possible etiological aspects of the disease. Its members were directed to ascertain whether the disease from which the prisoners of war were suffering was really Pellagra. They were also asked to investigate whether in general the prisoners were afflicted with the disease prior or subsequent to capture and whether the incidence of the disease was increasing, and if so, to explain how this came about: was it spreading by infection from person to person, was its spread facilitated by location or local conditions, and was it connected to diet. Finally, they were also asked to investigate the possible etiology of the disease in relation to bacteria, protozoa, blood conditions, pathology, and food.

The Committee was directed to begin work immediately and to submit its conclusions as soon as possible, which it did on 31 December 1918, less than three months after it had been appointed. During these weeks the committee had carried out a superb scientific and epidemiological task. Its main conclusions were that the disease under investigation was truly Pellagra, and that most of those ill with it had suffered from the disease prior to capture. There was no evidence of case-to-case infection or of infection due to location or local conditions. The committee found that Pellagra resulted from a deficiency of protein in the diet.

> A careful study of all available information reveals so constant an association between the biological protein value of diet and the occurrence of Pellagra, that the Committee considers that lack of sufficient biological value of protein stands in aetiological relation to Pellagra, certainly as an exciting factor and possibly as the determining factor.

The committee was unable to conclude whether this deficiency was absolute or relative, as regards the balance between energy income and expenditure and individual variations.[27] Its recommendations were all in the field of nutrition: to supply the prisoners of war a variety of food and meet any increase in the number of Pellagra cases by an increment of animal protein in the diet.

The recommendations were immediately implemented. The outcome was a steady decrease in the number of Pellagrins. Though no new cases were diagnosed among the Turkish prisoners of war, they were diagnosed among several workers belonging to the Egyptian Labour Corps and also among several German prisoners. They were treated according to the committee's recommendations and all recovered from the disease.

The professional reaction of the medical community to the committee's work, as reflected by an editorial article in the *British Medical Journal*, one of the leading medical journals in Britain at the time, was quite unique: 'The report of the Committee of Enquiry regarding the prevalence of Pellagra amongst Turkish prisoners of war will stand for years to come as a record of one of the best and most scientific inquiries ever accomplished by a nation at war.'[28]

In the meantime the pursuit of the retreating Turkish units continued. The 5th Cavalry Division troops rested at Homs for three days until the order came to advance on Aleppo, 120 miles to the north. The brigades began to move northwards in two columns, the first consisting of armoured cars, while the second included mainly mounted units. On 23 October an armoured car patrol approached Aleppo and observed the enemy entrenched south of the city. In an effort to avoid an unnecessary military encounter, the patrol commander was sent by Major-General H.J.M. Macandrew, commander of the 5th Cavalry Division, under a flag of truce, to demand the surrender of Aleppo. The demand was refused by the Turks. The armoured car column then awaited the arrival of the rest of the division. On 25 October the division's 15th Brigade arrived together with the Arab force. General Macandrew planned to attack the city from three directions on the morrow: the 15th Brigade from the west, the armoured column from the south, and the Arab force from the east. However, the Arabs entered the city during the night of the 25th, engaged in hand to hand fighting, and eventually reached the city's citadel. As a result, the Turks retreated from the city.

During the morning of 26 October the 15th Brigade moved west of Aleppo and gained control of the Aleppo–Alexandretta road several miles northwest of Aleppo. While Major-General Macandrew made his formal entrance into the city, the brigade was engaged in a battle against a retreating superior Turkish force near Haritan. The battle continued till dusk and was won when the 14th Brigade joined the 15th, causing the Turkish force to retreat. This was the last military engagement of the war in the Middle East theatre. The division sustained only few casualties during its entire advance of 250 miles.

On 31 October 1918 the exhausted Ottoman Empire signed a truce agreement with Britain and all hostilities ceased. On that same day General Allenby sent the CIGS in London his last despatch in which he described the EEF activities during the final stage of the campaign (19 September until 31October 1918). In the concluding paragraph he wrote:

> The rapid advance has rendered difficult the task of evacuating the sick and wounded. The difficulty was increased by the large number of prisoners who, after marching for days, with little food or water, surrendered in a state of extreme weakness, unable to march another day. The care and evacuation of these men has heavily taxed the Medical Services, who have worked untiringly.[29]

EPILOGUE

'Looking back now, with the experience of two wars in my mind, I think we learnt several things in Palestine which the men in France never learnt, and which were forgotten until the Second World War again thrust them upon us.'

J. Johnston Abraham, *Surgeon's Journey: The Autobiography of J. Johnston Abraham* (London: Heinemann, 1957), 244.

It was the end of November 1918. Most of the armistice agreements had already been signed and hostilities were over. Various units which had made up the multi-national mosaic of the EEF were, at last, on their way home. The New Zealanders, who had been in the Middle East from the beginning of the war, decided to pay a visit to Gallipoli. There, at the very place where many of their comrades had lost their lives on the battlefield, the Spanish Flue awaited them. The survivors of Gallipoli, the Sinai desert, and the Palestine campaigns were to fight their last battle, this time against a ruthless pandemic. One hundred and ten New Zealanders were evacuated to hospital due to their deteriorating medical condition, where eleven of them died. Most probably the last victims of disease during the Great War in the Middle East, they were buried near their comrades in the English Cemetery at Gallipoli.[1]

The British military forces now began to leave the Middle East. Field Marshall Allenby became Governor of Egypt, while Palestine would come under British Mandate. Colonel David Heron, RAMC, an expert in preventive medicine and diseases of the Middle East, would be appointed to head the

Health Department of the future British Mandate Government of Palestine. He would fill the same position for more than twenty years, doing a great job. When, in 1948, the British Mandate came to an end, Colonel Heron's Health Department served as a template for the Ministry of Health of the newly established State of Israel.

The anonymous heroes of this story – the sick and wounded soldiers and civilians, as well as the stretcher-bearers, medical orderlies, and Medical Officers – were now on their way home. Each of them carried with him his own experience of suffering and of the banality and intensity of war. Looking retrospectively, it seems that all these people who had sacrificed so much could do nothing to prevent future wars.

The medical heroes of the Palestine campaigns returned to their former lives. Richard H. Luce, the DMS EEF, the first territorial medical officer promoted during the war to be a surgeon general with the rank of Major General, returned to England and to his practice as a surgeon. For many years he served as a senior surgeon, and later a consulting surgeon, to the Derbyshire Royal Infirmary. Living in Derby, he became involved in local politics and was elected to Parliament in 1924, serving as a Member of Parliament for five years. Sir Richard also became interested in the history of his native town and wrote a classic book about the history of the old Benedictine Monastery at Malmesbury. He also wrote a book about the history of Romsey Abbey. In 1935 he was elected mayor of the town of Romsey and served the community for two years. He was highly respected as a surgeon and a human being. Sir Richard H. Luce died at the age of eighty-five in 1952.[2]

Rupert M. Downes, the DDMS of the Desert Mounted Corps, the bright, innovative, and creative medical officer who according to his commander General Harry Chauvel 'loved soldiering second only to medicine,'[3] remained in the military. He contributed much of his military experience to the education of medical officers and wrote several instructive professional articles concerning military medicine. He also wrote the medical history of the Desert Mounted Corps during the Palestine campaigns. Major General Rupert M. Downes of the 2nd Australian Army was killed in an air accident on 5 March 1945.

Surgeon and author Dr James Johnston Abraham, the efficient ADMS of Palestine L-of-C, returned to his surgical practice and became a prominent surgeon in London. He continued his literary work and was highly appreciated both as a surgeon and as a writer. He was in London during the Second World War air raids. In 1957 he published his autobiographical memoirs under the title *Surgeon's Journey*. In one of the most important chapters in this book Dr. Abraham tried to summarize the medical lessons of the Palestine campaigns as he understood them:

> Looking back now, with the experience of two wars in my mind, I think we learnt several things in Palestine which the men in France never learnt, and which were forgotten until the Second World War again thrust them upon us. One was the value of mobility. The Field Ambulances never got bogged down by unwieldy equipment. They moved with the troops. The Casualty Clearing Stations did not hold up the wounded. They sent them back as speedily as possible. We were the first to use planes to evacuate wounded. [...] The second thing we learnt was the value of expert surgery at the front. We had four surgical mobile units, [...] equipped with all the necessary tools for major surgery. They worked at the Main Dressing Stations of the Field Ambulances or at the nearest C.C.S., and were an innovation of immense importance. The third advance was the establishment of malaria diagnostic centres under Major Manson-Bahr [...], an advance which established a precedent which ought to have been of inestimable value in the Second World War.[4]

Were the medical lessons of the Palestine campaigns really important for the medical services treating the sick and wounded soldiers of future wars? Were the lessons of the Great War in general relevant to future wars? From the medical point of view, most of the weapons used then have changed for the worse, having a more detrimental effect on tissues and creating devastating injuries. Cavalry is only a distant memory of a more innocent world. Most of the medical evacuation of casualties from the front line is today performed by armoured vehicles and helicopters. Thus, one may conclude that the medical lessons of previous wars in general have no relevance for the present. That, however, is only partially true, as prevention of disease, coping with environmental and climatic hazards, and providing the best treatment as close to the firing line and as soon as possible are still essential on the modern battlefield. Good military medicine on the battlefield should always be performed in the tradition of the Palestine campaigns, where devotion, dedication, and professional excellence were its hallmarks.

NOTES

PROLOGUE

1. Thomas J. Mitchell and Georgie M. Smith, *Medical Services: Casualties and Medical Statistics of* the *Great War*, History of the Great War, Based on Official Documents (Nashville, TN: The Imperial War Museum and the Battery Press, 1997), 208–17. (Originally published: London: HMSO, 1931).
2. Michael Carver, *The Turkish Front, 1914–1918* (London: Sigdwick & Jackson in association with the National Army Museum, 2003), vii.

CHAPTER ONE

1. A well-written account of the organization of the RAMC during the Great War may be found in Thomas B. Nichols, *Organization, Strategy and Tactics of the Army Medical Services in War*, 2d ed. (London: Ballière, Tindall and Cox, 1940). For a general background concerning the history of military medicine before the First World War, see Fielding H. Garrison, *Notes on the History of Military Medicine* (Washington, DC: Association of Military Surgeons, 1922). About military medicine during the Great War, see Fred Smith, *A Short History of the Royal Army Medical Corps*, 2d ed. (Aldershot: Gale & Polden, 1931); Peter Lovegrove, *Not Least in the Crusade: A Short History of the Royal Army Medical Corps* (Aldershot: Gale & Polden, 1951); 'The Royal Army Medical Corps and Its Work,' *British Medical Journal* (1917), part II: 217–24.
2. Eran Dolev & Craig H. Llewellyn, 'The Chain of Medical Responsibility in Battlefield Medicine,' *Military Medicine* 150 (1985): 471–75.
3. 'The Medical Needs of the Army,' *British Medical Journal* (1915), part I: 511–12.
4. Nichols, *Organization, Strategy and Tactics*, 81–86.
5. Every Medical Officer used the 'Horrocks' Box' devised by Colonel Sir William Horrocks, RAMC, for water purification by chlorination.
6. The British Army infantry division comprised about 18,000 troops. It was formed of three infantry brigades and several other units (Royal Engineers, Artillery, RAMC, etc.). The infantry brigade consisted of four infantry battalions, each of which comprised four companies, with every company being made up of four platoons. An infantry battalion at

full strength consisted of 1,017 men; a battalion at 'full fighting strength' had 895 troops. Several divisions formed a Corps and several Corps an Army. A British cavalry division consisted of three cavalry brigades, each brigade having three cavalry regiments. A cavalry regiment was made up of 546 men and in 'full fighting strength' consisted of 510 cavalrymen. Thus, a British cavalry division with nine cavalry regiments consisted of about 8,000 men.

7. Ian R. Whitehead, *Doctors in the Great War* (Barnsley: L. Cooper, 1999), 184–86.
8. Sepsis, also known as septicemia, is the dissemination of micro-organisms from an infected wound into the blood stream. Even in the antibiotic era it carries a grave prognosis. Asepsis is a medical policy according to which any surgical procedure is performed in a sterile environment in order to prevent any contamination with germs. Antisepsis is a medical attitude which assumes that any injury is contaminated with germs and thus any treatment should include the use of antimicrobial solutions.
9. John S.G. Blair, *In Arduis Fidelis: Centenary History of the Royal Army Medical Corps* (Edinburgh: Scottish Academic Press, 1998), 19.
10. Nichols, *Organization, Strategy and Tactics*, 113–20. The medical equipment of the field ambulance was carried in 'panniers,' canvas skips, especially designed for this purpose.
11. Henry M.W. Gray, *The Early Treatment of War Wounds* (London: Hodder & Stoughton, 1919), 49–50.
12. Nichols, *Organization, Strategy and Tactics*, 87–97.
13. Ibid., 98–106.
14. Arthur G. Butler, *The Official History of the Australian Army Medical Services in the War of 1914–18*, vol. 1: *Gallipoli, Palestine and New Guinea* (Melbourne: Australian War Memorial, 1938), 830–31.
15. Ibid., 591 n. 4.
16. Ibid., 643–43.
17. Edward H. Benton, 'British Surgery in the South African War,' *Medical History* 21 (1977): 275–90; William MacCormac, 'Some Remarks, by Way of Contrast on War Surgery, Old and New,' *British Medical Journal* (1901) part II: 459–62; George H. Makins, *Surgical Experiences in South Africa 1899–1900: Being Mainly a Clinical Study of the Nature and Effects of Injuries Produced by Bullets of Small Calibre*, 2d ed. (London: Hodder & Stoughton, 1913); David B. Adams, 'Abdominal Gunshot Wounds in Warfare: a Historical Review,' *Military Medicine* 148 (1983): 15–20.
18. Cuthbert Wallace, 'War Surgery of the Abdomen, Part I,' *Lancet* (1917) part I: 561–68.
19. Blair, *In Arduis Fidelis*, 74.
20. Ibid., 75. Laparotomy is the surgical procedure by which the abdomen is opened and explored.
21. Benton, 'British Surgery.'
22. Whitehead, *Doctors in the Great War*, 164; George H. Makins, 'The Role of the Consulting Surgeon in War,' *Lancet* (1919) part I: 1099–1102; 'Consultants with the Army Abroad,' *British Medical Journal* (1919) part I: 804–5.
23. Peter K. Bamberger, 'The Adoption of Laparotomy for the Treatment of Penetrating Abdominal Wounds in War,' *Military Medicine* 161 (1996): 189–96.
24. Blair, *In Arduis Fidelis*, 169.
25. *Medical Services: Surgery of the War*, eds. William G. Macpherson, Anthony A. Bowlby, Cuthbert S. Wallace, and Thomas C. English, 2 vols., History of the Great War, Based on Official Documents (London: HMSO, 1922), 1:211; 'British Surgery at the Front,' *British Medical Journal* (1917) part I: 137; Anthony A. Bowlby, 'British Military Surgery in the Time of Hunter and in the Great War,' *British Medical Journal* (1917) part I: 737.

26. A.H. Stafford, 'Casualty Clearing Station,' *Military Surgeon* 48 (1921): 334–40.
27. 'The Royal Army Medical Corps and Its Work': 254–60; *Medical Services: Surgery of the War*, 1:211–16.
28. Thomas H. Goodwin, 'The Collection and Evacuation of Sick and Wounded from Front to Base,' *Military Surgeon* 40 (1917): 609–19.
29. Bowlby, 'British Military Surgery.'
30. Butler, *Official History*, 832.
31. Thomas H. Goodwin, 'The Organization and Administration of the British Army with Especial Reference to the Medical Services,' *Military Surgeon* 41 (1917): 32–42; H. Ensor, 'The R.A.M.C. Services of a Division on Active Service,' *Journal of the Royal Army Medical Corps* 42 (1924): 241–58, 331–43, 424–37.
32. Nichols, *Organization, Strategy and Tactics*, 253–55.
33. Ibid., 271–72.
34. John Gilmour, 'Transportation of Wounded,' *Military Surgeon* 42 (1918): 1–12.
35. Nichols, *Organization, Strategy and Tactics*, 205–6.
36. Gilmour, 'Transportation of Wounded.'
37. *Medical Services: Surgery of the War*, 2:310.
38. Rupert M. Downer, 'The Tactical Employment of the Medical Services in a Cavalry Corps,' *Journal of the Royal Army Medical Corps*', 47 (1926): 328–34.

CHAPTER TWO

1. Archibald P. Wavell, *The Palestine Campaigns*, 3d ed. (London: Constable, 1932), 25.
2. Ibid., 27.
3. George F. MacMunn and Cyril Falls, *Military Operations Egypt & Palestine: From the Outbreak of War with Germany to June 1917*, History of the Great War Based on Official Documents (London: HMSO, 1928), 1:368–69.
4. Freiherr Friedrich Kress von Kressenstein, *Mit den Türken zum Suezkanal* (Berlin: O. Schlegel, 1938).
5. There is a vast literature concerning the campaign in the Dardanelles. The following is a basic list that includes mainly references which deal with or emphasize the medical aspects of the campaign: Mitchell and Smith, *Medical Services: Casualties and Medical Statistics*, 198–207; Michael B. Tyquin, *Gallipoli, the Medical War: The Australian Army Medical Services in the Dardanelles Campaign of 1915* (Kensington, Australia: New South Wales University Press, 1993); Robert Rhodes James, *Gallipoli* (London: Pimlico, 1999); Nigel Steel and Peter Hart, *Defeat at Gallipoli* (London: Macmillan, 1994); 'A Medical View of the Gallipoli Adventure,' *Lancet* (1916) part I: 141–42; 'Dysentery at Gallipoli,' *British Medical Journal* (1917) part I: 738–39; E.L. Atkinson, 'The Fly Pest in Gallipoli,' *Journal of the Royal Naval Medical Service* 2 (1916): 147–50.
6. For several aspects of the campaign in Mesopotamia, see Ronald W. Millar, *Death of an Army: The Siege of Kut 1915–1916* (Boston: Houghton Mifflin, 1970); Anthony J. Barker, *The Bastard War: The Mesopotamian Campaign of 1914–1918* (New York: Dial Press, 1967); Russell Braddon, *The Siege* (New York: Viking Press, 1970); Charles V.F. Townshend, *My Campaigns in Mesopotamia* (London: Thornton Butterworth, 1920); 'The Mesopotamia Report,' *Lancet* (1917) part II: 17.
7. MacMunn and Falls, *Military Operations […] from the Outbreak of War with Germany to June 1917*, 170–74; Wavell, *Palestine Campaigns*, 41–42.
8. Wavell, *Palestine Campaigns*, 92.

9. William G. Macpherson, *Medical Services: General History*, History of the Great War Based on Official Documents, 4 vols. (London: HMSO, 1921–24), 3:413.
10. Ibid., 411–12.
11. Ibid., 4:598–603.
12. MacMunn and Falls, *Military Operations [...] from the Outbreak of War with Germany to June 1917*, 204 n. 4: The evacuation of the wounded; Macpherson, *Medical Services: General History*, 4:615–17.
13. Macpherson, *Medical Services: General History*, 4:604.
14. 'Larrie,' 'Concerning Medical Blokes,' in *Australia in Palestine*, eds. Henry S. Gullett and Charles L. Barrett (Sydney: Angus and Robertson, 1919), 103.
15. Butler, *Official History*, 475.
16. Ibid., 482. According to Desert Column Order No. 20, Chapter 11, 'Training of Medical Units in Real Scenario" issued on 3 July 1916, PRO WO 95/4429: Ambulance Convoy to operate between mobile and immobile sections of the field ambulance to include: 2 horses, 32 mules, 71 camels, 16 fanatis, 32 cacolets, 8 sand carts. Every mobile section of a field ambulance has the means to evacuate at one time: 46 lying and 68 sitting casualties. This is available with: 42 stretchers, 68 cacolets, 2 sand carts.
17. MacMunn and Falls, *Military Operations [...] from the Outbreak of War with Germany to June 1917*, 199.
18. Wavell, *Palestine Campaigns*, 57.
19. MacMunn and Falls, *Military Operations [...] from the Outbreak of War with Germany to June 1917*, 251. A 'railhead' was 'a locality on the railway where ammunition and supplies were, at the nearest point to the force to be served' (Butler, *Official History*, 834).
20. Macpherson, *Medical Services: General History*, 3:416–17.
21. Ibid., 3:419.
22. Ibid.
23. Wavell, *Palestine Campaigns*, 58.
24. Butler, *Official History*, 591.
25. Alexander H.C. Kearsey, *The Operations in Egypt and Palestine*, 3d ed. (Aldershot: Gale & Polden, 1937), 43; Macpherson, *Medical Services: General History*, 3:421.
26. Butler, *Official History*, 591.
27. Henry S. Gullett, *The Australian Imperial Force in Sinai and Palestine, 1914–1918*, The Official History of Australia in the War of 1914–1918; v. 7 (Sydney: Angus & Robertson, 1923), 457.
28. Butler, *Official History*, 592–93; Anderson D. Carbery, *The New Zealand Medical Service in the Great War, 1914–1918, Based on Official Documents* (Auckland: Whitcombe & Tombs, 1924), 457.
29. Macpherson, *Medical Services: General History*, 3:422.
30. Charles G. Powles, *The New Zealanders in Sinai and Palestine*, Official History of New Zealand's Effort in the Great War; v. 3 (Auckland: Whitcombe & Tombs, 1922), 78.
31. Eran Dolev, 'The First Recorded Aeromedical Evacuation in the British Army – the True Story,' *Journal of the Royal Army Medical Corps* 132 (1986): 34–36; the event is also mentioned in the diary of the Imperial Camel Corps, PRO WO 95/4403.
32. Sir Archibald Murray wrote in his last despatch: 'The health of the troops has throughout been singularly good. All branches of the medical services, under Surgeon General J. Maher, C.B., deserve the highest commendation for their successful work at the front, on the Lines of Communication and in the base hospitals. The presence in the force of a number of civil medical consultants, who have so patriotically given their services, has been of the very greatest value, and they have worked in successful accord with the regular medical

services of the Army. The Australian Army Medical Corps and the New Zealand Medical Corps have also been remarkable for their efficiency and unremitting devotion.' Archibald Murray, *Despatches*, 2 vols. (London: J.M. Dent & Sons, 1920), 2:174.

33. Mark Harrison, 'The British Army and the Problem of Venereal Disease in France and Egypt during the First World War,' *Medical History* 39 (1995): 133–58.
34. Ion L. Idriess, *The Desert Column: Leaves from the Diary of an Australian Trooper in Gallipoli, Sinai and Palestine* (Sydney: Angus & Robertson, 1932), 137–38; ADMS, 52nd Division, 'Brief Report on the Outbreak of Cholera Occurring among the Units of No. 3 Section, Canal defences,' 4 Aug. 1916, PRO WO 95/4598; diary of the EEF DMS, 31 Aug. 1916, PRO WO 95/4387. A suspected cholera outbreak occurred at Port Said. A real cholera epidemic broke out at Akaba on 18 Oct. 1917. It seemed at the time to be such a threat that an RAMC officer, Captain Willmore, was sent especially from Cairo to investigate this outbreak, arriving a week later, on 25 Oct. 1917. The event was mentioned in the diary of the DQMG (Deputy Quartermaster General), PRO WO 95/4380.
35. Macpherson, *Medical Services: General History*, 3:433–34.
36. Diary of the Director of Supply and Transport, EEF, 26 Dec. 1916, PRO WO 95/4395.
37. Macpherson, *Medical Services: General History*, 3:434; H. Warren Crowe, 'A Routine Treatment for Septic Sores and Nile Boils,' *Lancet* (1918) part II: 667–69; Antony Bluett, *With Our Army in Palestine* (London: Melrose, 1919), 24.
38. MacMunn and Falls, *Military Operations [...] from the Outbreak of War with Germany to June 1917*, 281.
39. Diary notation of Major W.S. Scott, 15 Apr. 1917, IWM 99/12/1.
40. Wavell, *Palestine Campaigns*, 80; Butler, *Official History*, 620.
41. OC Desert Column, Order 25, chapter 6, 25 Mar. 1917, PRO WO 95/4549.
42. *Medical Services: Surgery of the War*, 1:311.
43. J. Johnston Abraham, *Surgeon's Journey: the Autobiography of J. Johnston Abraham* (London: Heinemann, 1957), 179.
44. Memoir of Captain P.C. Duncan, the 2nd/4th Queen's Own Battalion, the 53rd Division, 9–10, IWM 79/51/1.
45. Idriess, *Desert Column*, 208.
46. Oskar Teichman, *The Diary of a Yeomanry M.O.: Egypt, Gallipoli, Palestine and Italy* (London: T. Fisher Unwin, 1921), 146.
47. Bluett, *With Our Army in Palestine*, 130–31.
48. Yigal Sheffy, 'Chemical Warfare and the Palestine Campaign in World War I,' *Cathedra* 105 (Sept. 2002): 41–84 (Hebrew); General Dobbel's plan for 'Second Gaza,' 7 Apr. 1917 (E.S. 125), PRO WO 95/4450; 17 Apr. 1917, ibid.; 52nd Division Standing Order No. 4: 'Gas Attack,' 13 Apr. 1917, PRO WO 95/4597. 'Our second great enterprise, gas, was a failure too. The atmosphere seems to dissolve the gas immediately the shells explode' (Idriess, *Desert Column*, 201).
49. Diary of the ANZAC Mounted Division, PRO WO 95/4549 and PRO WO 95/4523.
50. *Medical Services: Surgery of the War*, 1:311–12.
51. Wavell, *Palestine Campaigns*, 88; Butler, *Official History*, 622.
52. Abraham, *Surgeon's Journey*, 179–80.
53. Ibid., 178.
54. Ibid., 189–90.
55. Fourth despatch, 28 June 1917, Murray, *Despatches*, 164.
56. MacMunn and Falls, *Military Operations [...] from the Outbreak of War with Germany to June 1917*, 355.
57. Ibid., 358. General Bulfin was later promoted by Allenby to OC of the XXI Corps. He

was succeeded on 7 August 1917 by Major General J.S.M. Shea, who would distinguish himself as the division's commander throughout the Palestine campaigns.

58. Ibid., 358.
59. Ibid., 368.

CHAPTER THREE

1. Lawrence James, *Imperial Warrior: the Life and Times of Field-Marshal Viscount Allenby 1861–1936* (London: Weidenfeld and Nicolson, 1993), 106.
2. Basil H. Liddell-Hart, 'Allenby,' in *Famous British Generals*, eds. Barrett Watson [et al.] (London: Nicolson & Watson, 1951), 130.
3. Ibid., 119.
4. Archibald P. Wavell, *Allenby: A Study in Greatness: The Biography of Field-Marsal Viscount Allenby of Megiddo and Felixstowe* (London: G. Harrap, 1940), 87, 99–100.
5. Ibid., 112–13.
6. For the relations between Haig and Allenby during their studies at the Staff College, see ibid., 61–63; for their relations during the war, see 170, 183–84.
7. Liddell-Hart, 'Allenby,' 138.
8. Ibid., 131.
9. Kenneth Macksey, *The Shadow of Vimy Ridge* (London: W. Kimber, 1965), 56–57; Liddell-Hart, 'Allenby,' 119.
10. Anthony Farrar-Hockley, 'Field Marshal the Viscount Allenby,' in *The War Lords: Military Commanders of the Twentieth Century*, ed. Michael Carver (London: Weidenfeld and Nicolson, 1976), 144–59.
11. Matthew Hughes, *Allenby and British Strategy in the Middle East, 1917–1919* (London: F. Cass, 1999), 2, 9.
12. Jonathan Newell, 'Allenby and the Palestine Campaign,' in *The First World War and British Military History*, ed. Brian Bond (Oxford: Clarendon Press, 1991), 203.
13. Wavell, *Allenby*, 179–80.
14. Jonathan Newell, 'Learning the Hard Way: Allenby in Egypt and Palestine 1917–1919,' *Journal of Strategic Studies* 14 (1991): 363–87.
15. Wavell, *Allenby*, 62.
16. Ibid., 91–92.
17. James, *Imperial Warrior*, 22.
18. Raymond Savage, *Allenby of Armageddon: A Record of the Career and Campaigns of Field-Marshal Viscount Allenby G.C.B. G.C.M.G.* (London: Hodder and Stoughton, 1925), 199; James, *Imperial Warrior*, 82.
19. George de Symons Barrow, *The Fire of Life* (London: Hutchinson, 1942), 46.
20. Wavell, *Allenby*, 187; Brian Gardner, *Allenby* (London: Cassell, 1965), 164.
21. James, *Imperial Warrior*, 234.
22. Wavell, *Allenby*, 166.
23. *The War the Infantry Knew: A Chronicle of Service [...] Founded on Personal Records, Recollections and Reflections, Assembled, Edited and Partly Written by One of Their Medical Officers* [=James C. Dunn] (London: Jane's, 1987), 358.
24. Wavell, *Allenby*, 299.
25. Ibid., 185–89.
26. Ibid., 236; LHMCA, Allenby Papers, 1/7/1.
27. Wavell, *Allenby*, 35.

28. Ibid., 38.
29. Ibid., 169, 257.
30. Ibid., 120.
31. Ibid., 111–12; James, *Imperial Warrior*, 116.
32. Wavell, *Allenby*, 168–69; Savage, *Allenby of Armageddon*, 49, 133, 144–45; Gardner, *Allenby*, 148.
33. Hughes, *Allenby and British Strategy*, 23–42.
34. Abraham, *Surgeon's Journey*, 161, 190.
35. John N. More, *With Allenby's Crusaders* (London: Heath, Cranton, 1923), 57.
36. Alec J. Hill, *Chauvel of the Light Horse: A Biography of General Sir Harry Chauvel, G.C.M.G., K.C.B.* (Carlton, Vic.: Melbourne University Press, 1978), 133–34.
37. Alfred H. Tubby, *A Consulting Surgeon in the Near East* (London: Christophers, 1920), 192–93.
38. Thomas E. Lawrence, *Seven Pillars of Wisdom*, Wordsworth Classics of World Literature (Hertfordshire: Wordsworth Editions, 1997), chap. CXXII, 654–55.
39. James Barrett, 'The Halford Oration,' *Medical Journal of Australia* (1932) part II: 707–18. Delivered on 23 Nov. 1932.
40. Geoffrey Inchbald, *Imperial Camel Corps* (London: Johnson, 1970), 126–27.
41. Wavell, *Allenby*, 168.
42. From a letter written by Major General Sir Richard H. Luce, Surgeon General of the EEF during the last phase of the Palestine campaign, to General Wavell, 1 December 1936; LHMCA, Allenby Papers, 1/6/8.
43. Ibid.
44. Ibid.
45. Letter no. 8715, 14 Dec. 1917, LHMCA, Allenby Papers, 2/5/6.
46. LHMCA, Allenby Papers, 1/1/2.
47. Savage, *Allenby of Armageddon*, 134, 149.
48. Chetwode to Wavell, LHMCA, Allenby Papers, 1/6/8.
49. Gardner, *Allenby*, 126. Rupert Brooke (1887–1915) died from what was defined at the time as 'blood poisoning' on his way to Gallipoli.
50. Ibid., 148.
51. Ibid., 164.
52. Wavell, *Allenby*, 257.

CHAPTER FOUR

1. A letter of Lance Corporal Loudon, the 52nd Division, IWM, Document no. 87/17/1.
2. Abraham, *Surgeon's Journey*, 190.
3. Butler, *Official History*, 627–28.
4. Allenby to CIGS, IWM, Document no. 01/3(569).42/319; Telegram E.A.40, 12 July 1917, chapter 9, PRO WO 95/4367.
5. Wavell, *Allenby*, 203.
6. See Chapter 6 below.
7. Wavell, *Palestine Campaigns*, 241; Yigal Sheffy, 'The Origins of the British Breakthrough into South Palestine: The ANZAC Raid on the Ottoman Railway, 1917,' *Journal of Strategic Studies* 22 (1999): 124–47.
8. 'Appreciaton of the Situation,' 17 June 1917, IWM, Dawnay Papers, 69/21/2.
9. Abraham, *Surgeon's Journey*, 178.

10. 'Notes for D.M.O. and C.I.G.S. on Plan of Operations, Palestine Front' issued by Lt Colonel A.P. Wavell, General Staff, HQ EEF, 15 Aug. 1917, PRO WO 106/725.
11. Diary of Major W.S. Scott,, IWM, Document no. 99/12/1; Order for the attack against Beersheba, 22 Oct. 1917, PRO WO 95/4521–22; *The Work of the Royal Engineers in the World War, 1914-19: Work in the Field in Other Theatres of War, Egypt and Palestine,* vol. [2]: *Water-supply.* (Chatham: Published by the Secretary, Institution of the Royal Engineers; W. & J. Mackay & Co., 1921), 31.
12. Sheffy, 'Chemical Warfare.'
13. Diary of Col. A.E.C. Keble, EEF DMS, PRO WO 95/4386.
14. *Medical Services: Surgery of the War*, 2:312–13.
15. Butler, *Official History*, 663 n. 1.
16. 'Medical Arrangements,' in Appendix G of the administrative plan for the future operation, written by Colonel Luce, DDMS XX Corps, 30 Sept. 1917, PRO WO 95/4483.
17. Richard H. Luce, 'War Experiences of a Territorial Medical Officer,' 474. The original memoir was published in the form of consecutive chapters in the *Journal of the Royal Army Medical Corps*, between April 1936 and December 1937, mainly in volume 46. The memoirs were then collected and bound; the document, with the same title, is deposited in WIHM CAMC/RAMC, document No. 2031.
18. Abraham, *Surgeon's Journey*, 196–98.
19. Ralph E.C. Adams, *The Modern Crusaders* (London: Routledge & Sons, 1920), 28.
20. Luce, 'War Experiences,' 469.
21. Medical arrangements for the future operations, written by Colonel C.J. Macdonald, DDMS XXI Corps, 16 Oct. 1917, PRO WO 95/4490; Order of the ANZAC Mounted Division; section No. 12 describes the medical arrangements, 27 Oct. 1917, PRO WO 95/4522.
22. 'Wire roads' were a special device used while advancing in deserts and deep sandy terrain. These were metal nets laid out along a route to prevent vehicles from sinking in the sand. Dr J.J. Abraham wrote: 'Some genius has just invented the wire road. This was made of two six-feet-wide rolls of rabbit-wire netting laid on the sand and pegged down to make a twelve-foot track. On this we could run an ambulance car.' (Abraham, *Surgeon's Journey*, 169).
23. Order No. 38, 17 Oct. 1917, PRO WO 95/4368.
24. Luce, 'War Experiences,' 466.
25. Acting Sgt J.E. Scott, 2nd London Sanitary Company, RAMC, IWM, Document no. 79/1/1.
26. *Medical Services: Surgery of the War*, 2:313. The French Medical Services had been using the Boulant Mobile Surgery Unit since 1912. This was a motor vehicle which contained an operating theatre, a water tank, and a sterilization unit and was ready for tenting. Its speed was 30 km/hr and was considered too expensive. See Chris Ellis, *Military Transport of World War I: Including Vintage Vehicles and Post War Models* (London: Blandford Press, 1970), 134.
27. Carbery, *New Zealand Medical Service*, 466.
28. Butler, *Official History*, 664 n. 1.
29. Teichman, *Diary of a Yeomanry M.O.*, 11–15.
30. 'Musketeer,' 'The Memoirs of a Professional Soldier in Peace and War' (typescript, dated 29 Apr. 1968), 19, LHCMA, Clarke 1/1. 'Musketeer' is Major Clarke, who served at the time in the 162nd Brigade of the 54th (East Anglian) Division.
31. Captain P.C. Duncan, 53rd Division, IWM, Document no. 79/51/1, 11–12.
32. Eran Dolev, 'Captain John Fox Russell, V.C., M.C., R.A.M.C. (1893–1917): A Forgot-

ten Hero of Military Medicine,' *Journal of the Royal Army Medical Corps* 142 (1996): 126–28.

33. 'Scheme of Medical Arrangements for Forthcoming Operation of XXth Corps,' PRO WO 95/ 4483; Diary of Col. A.E.C. Keble, EEF DMS, PRO WO 95/4386; Diary of CCS No. 35, PRO WO 95/4733.
34. LHCMA, Allenby Papers, 1/4.

CHAPTER FIVE

1. Teichman, *Diary of a Yeomanry M.O.*, 185.
2. Abraham, *Surgeon's Journey*, 171; Cyril Falls, *Military Operations, Egypt & Palestine: From June 1917 to the End of the War,* History of the Great War Based on Official Documents, 2 vols. (London: HMSO, 1930), 1:144.
3. Abraham, *Surgeon's Journey*, 203.
4. Falls, *Military Operations [...] from June 1917 to the End of the War*, 1:129.
5. Teichman, *Diary of a Yeomanry M.O.*, 187–88.
6. H.F. Humphreys, 'Diary of a DADMS on the Jerusalem Campaign, Palestine, November-December 1917,' *Journal of the Royal Army Medical Corps* 50 (1928): 175–83.
7. Falls, *Military Operations [...] from June 1917 to the End of the War*, 1:164.
8. Carbery, *New Zealand Medical Service*, 469.
9. Ibid., 468–69.
10. Abraham, *Surgeon's Journey*, 205–6.
11. Butler, *Official History*, 672.
12. Carbery, *New Zealand Medical Service*, 469.
13. Philip H. Dalbiac, *History of the 60th Division (2/2nd London Division)* (London: George Allen & Unwin, 1927), 174.
14. J.L. Gray (Donald Black), *Red Dust: An Australian Trooper in Palestine* (London: Jonathan Cape, 1931), 94.
15. A document written by the BGGS, XXI Corps, analyzing the statistics of casualties of the infantry units during recent engagements, a chapter of the XXI Corps report of the operations during the advance to Jerusalem, 12 Jan. 1918, PRO WO95/4490.
16. Abraham, *Surgeon's Journey*, 203.
17. Ibid., 205.
18. 'Medical Arrangements – 75th Division, from 16th November–31st December, 1917'; Appendix 2 to XXI Corps report (n. 15 above), PRO WO95/4490.
19. Ibid.; Humphreys, 'Diary of a DADMS': 252–60.
20. Dalbiac, *History of the 60th Division*, 174–75.
21. Gray, *Red Dust*, 122–24.
22. Dalbiac, *History of the 60th Division*, 174.
23. Humphreys, 'Diary of a DADMS': 260.
24. Macpherson, *Medical Services: General History*, 3:449.
25. Ibid., 3:455–56.
26. Gardner, *Allenby*, 156.
27. Chetwode to Wavell, 28 Mar. 1939, LHMCA, Allenby Papers, 6/9.
28. Luce, 'War Experiences,' 494.
29. Dalbiac, *History of the 60th Division*, 175.
30. Captain Masta Mohammed of the 18th Turkish Infantry Brigade was killed on the road from Jerusalem on 18 Dec. 1917. IWM, MISC 168, item no. 2584.

31. Adams, *Modern Crusaders*; Wilfred S. Kent Hughes, *Modern Crusaders: An Account of the Campaign in Sinai and Palestine up to the Capture of Jerusalem* (Melbourne: Melville & Mullen, [1918]); Cecil Sommers, *Temporary Crusaders* (London: John Lane, 1918); More, *With Allenby's Crusaders*; Donald Maxwell, *The Last Crusade* (London: John Lane, 1920). These are only a few of the books which appeared during Allenby's lifetime whose title included the word 'Crusade'. This motif may be found in many of the publications which have described the Palestine campaigns.
32. EEF GHQ, Operations, 9 Dec. 1917, PRO WO95/4369.
33. Ernest W.G. Masterman, 'Jerusalem from the Point of View of Health and Disease,' *Lancet* (1918) part I: 305–7.
34. Raphael de Nogales, *Four Years beneath the Crescent*, trans. by M. Lee (London: Charles Scribner's Sons, 1926), 271.
35. Masterman, 'Jerusalem from the Point of View of Health and Disease.'
36. Perez Yekutiel, 'Masterman, Muehlens and Malaria, Jerusalem 1912–1913,' *Korot* 12 (1996): 107–23; Nogales, *Four Years*, 271.
37. William Canton, *Dawn in Palestine* (New York: Macmillan, 1918), 91.
38. Nogales, *Four Years*, 271–2.
39. Gray, *Red Dust*, 129.
40. Diary of DMS EEF, PRO WO95/4386.
41. Ya'akov Gross, *Jerusalem 1917/8* (Jerusalem: Koresh Publishers, 1992), 416–21 (Hebrew); Gray, *Red Dust*, 79–81.
42. Gross, *Jerusalem 1917/8*, 416–21.
43. EEF GHQ, Director of supplies and transport, 9 Dec. 1917, PRO WO95/4397.
44. Abraham, *Surgeon's Journey*, 208.
45. Ibid., 207.
46. Falls, *Military Operations [...] from June 1917 to the End of the War*, 1:264.
47. Dalbiac, *History of the 60th Division*, 177.

CHAPTER SIX

1. Allenby to Robertson, 23 Feb. 1918, LHCMA, Robertson Papers, 7/5/86. Cited in *Allenby in Palestine: The Middle East Correspondence of Field Marshal Viscount Allenby, June 1917–October 1919*, edited and selected by Mathew Hughes, Publications of the Army Records Society, vol. 22 (Stroud: Sutton, 2004), letter No 99, p. 133. There is no evidence concerning a special prevalence of typhus in Jericho.
2. William Travers Swan was born 28 September 1861. He served in India (Chitral) and then in the Boer War. In 1914 he was appointed ADMS 7th Division and then ADMS 5th Division. In July 1915 he was appointed DDMS VII Corps, 3rd Army, where he served under General Allenby. On 29 January 1918 he arrived at Alexandria and on 7 February in Palestine.
3. Liddell-Hart, 'Allenby,' 135.
4. 'The two raids to Salt had fixed the Turks' eyes exclusively beyond Jordan. Every move there, whether of British or Arabs, was accompanied by counter-precautions on the Turks' part, showing how fearful they were.' Lawrence, *Seven Pillars of Wisdom*, Chap. XCVIII, 535.
5. Gullett, *Australian Imperial Force*, 547; Hill, *Chauvel of the Light Horse*, 151; Chauvel to Wavell, 13 Oct. 1936, LHCMA, Allenby Papers 6/9.
6. Chetwode to Wavell, 28 Mar. 1939, LHCMA, Allenby Papers, 6/9.
7. For a very good description concerning the political background in the Middle East see

the writings of Prof. Elie Kedourie: *In the Anglo-Arab Labyrinth: The McMahon–Husayn Correspondence and Its Interpretations, 1914–1939* (Cambridge: Cambridge University Press, 1976); *England and the Middle East: The Destruction of the Ottoman Empire, 1914–1921* (London: Bowes & Bowes, 1956). The Balfour Declaration was delivered on 2 November 1917.

8. For concise background information, see *An Encyclopedia of World History*, ed. W.L. Langer, 6th ed. rev. and expanded, general ed. Peter N. Stearns (Boston: Houghton Mifflin, 2001), 937–38. The terms of the Sykes–Picot Treaty stipulated that Britain was to administrate the areas of the future states of Jordan and Iraq, while France would administrate the future areas of Syria, Lebanon, and North Iraq. Palestine was to be under international rule.
9. See Chapter 4.
10. There is a vast literature concerning T.E. Lawrence ('Lawrence of Arabia' 1888–1935) and his deeds. The best history and descriptions of the Arab Revolt were written by Lawrence himself: *Seven Pillars of Wisdom*, Wordsworth Classics of World Literature (Hertfordshire: Wordsworth Editions, 1997); *Revolt in the Desert* (Garden City, NY: Doubleday, Doran & Co., 1926). There were many myths and speculations concerning relations between Allenby and Lawrence. Again, it seems that the best source might be Lawrence himself: 'Allenby was physically large and confident, and morally so great' *Seven Pillars of Wisdom*; Chapter LVI, 323; '"Well, I will do for you what I can" and that ended it.[...] –but we learned gradually that he meant exactly what he said; and that what General Allenby could do was enough for his greediest servant' (ibid., 324). See also Jeremy Wilson, *Lawrence of Arabia: The Authorized Biography of T.E. Lawrence* (London: Minerva, 1990).
11. Wavell, *Palestine Campaigns*, 179.
12. Allenby to Robertson, 25 Jan. 1918, LHCMA, Robertson Papers, No. 7/5/84. Also Letter No. 94 in *Allenby in Palestine*, ed. Hughes, 127.
13. Falls, *Military Operations [...] from June 1917 to the End of the War*, 1:329.
14. A pontoon bridge was a floating bridge to enable crossing over narrow rivers or canals. It was made of boats arranged in a row, one alongside the other, across the river or canal, to serve as a basis for platforms over which the forces would cross.
15. Falls, *Military Operations [...] from June 1917 to the End of the War*, Appendix 20, 2: 705–6.
16. Dalbiac, *History of the 60th Division*, 207.
17. Luce, 'War Experiences,' 521.
18. Dalbiac, *History of the 60th Division*, 208–9.
19. Allenby to Robertson, 31 Mar. 1918, PRO WO 33/946, p. 312. Cited as letter No. 107 in *Allenby in Palestine*, ed. Hughes, 140.
20. Gullett, *Australian Imperial Force*, 577.
21. Butler, *Official History*, 684.
22. Gullett, *Australian Imperial Force*, 578.
23. Dalbiac, *History of the 60th Division*, 208–9.
24. Richard M.P. Preston, *The Desert Mounted Corps: An Account of the Cavalry Operations in Palestine and Syria1917–1918* (London: Constable, 1921), 152.
25. Dalbiac, *History of the 60th Division*, 210.
26. Allenby to War Office, 26 Apr. 1918, PRO WO 33/946; also Letter No. 114 in *Allenby in Palestine*, ed. Hughes, 145.
27. The German 'Ludendorf Offensive,' also known as the 'Great March Offensive,' was well planned and took the British by surprise. It began on 21 March with a massive bombardment and a heavy gas attack. In a few days the Germans drove back the British line about forty

miles. With the help of the French, this offensive was checked and lost its momentum. It was over by 5 April 1918.

28. Wavell, *Palestine Campaigns*, 189.
29. Falls, *Military Operations [...] from June 1917 to the End of the War*, 1:364–65.
30. Gullett, *Australian Imperial Force*, 622.
31. Falls, *Military Operations [...] from June 1917 to the End of the War*, 1:377.
32. Redcliffe N. Salaman, *Palestine Reclaimed: Letters from a Jewish Officer in Palestine* (London: G. Routledge, 1920), 85–86.
33. Hill, *Chauvel of the Light Horse*, 67.
34. Butler, *Official History*, 693–94 n. 7.
35. Preston, *Desert Mounted Corps*, 173; XX Corps HQ, 4 May 1918, PRO WO 95/4475: 'The total number of evacuations during these operations was 1784, of whom 1076 (including 310 from the Mounted Brigades) were wounded and 708 sick.' According to Falls, *Military Operations [...] from June 1917 to the End of the War*, 1:389: 'The number of British casualties was 1649.' In a footnote on that same page: 'Of these casualties 1116 [about two thirds of the whole] were incurred by the 60th Division and attached Patiala Infantry.'
36. LHCMA, Allenby Papers, 6/9.
37. Butler, *Official History*, 695.
38. Falls, *Military Operations [...] from June 1917 to the End of the War*, 1:392.

CHAPTER SEVEN

1. Butler, *Official History*, 698.
2. Major R.H.Wilson of the Berkshire Yeomanry, 13th Mounted Brigade, 5th Cavalry Division, The Desert Mounted Corps, IWM, Document no. 82/25/1.
3. Preston, *Desert Mounted Corps*, 181.
4. Gullett, *Australian Imperial Force*, 646; Wavell, *Allenby*, 257.
5. P. Manson-Bahr, 'Experiences in Malaria in the Egyptian Expeditionary Force,' *Lancet* (1920) part I: 79–85.
6. 'Malaria in the Armies,' *British Medical Journal* (1918) part I: 350–51.
7. A very important source which enables one to gain an understanding of the various attitudes towards malaria at the time of the Great War is William G. Willoughby and Louis L. Cassidy, *Anti-malaria Work in Macedonia among British Troops* (London: H.K. Lewis, 1918). It is interesting to compare it with the following quotations from another work: 'Had it from the first been possible to decide that in Macedonia protection from malaria was, after food and ammunition, the very first necessity, it is reasonable to suppose that the Salonika Army might have been kept at a higher standard of strength and efficiency, that a certain number of lives might have been saved, and that many thousands of men might have been spared ill health after the war.' 'In building up a striking force, an enormous wastage from malaria, a certain proportion of which was permanent wastage, had to be taken into account.' Cyril Falls, *Military Operations, Macedonia*, 2 vols. (London: HMSO, 1933–35), 1:288 and 2:294 respectively.
8. Gray, *Red Dust*, 161–62.
9. 'Koolawarra,' 'Malaria,' in *Australia in Palestine*, 144.
10. Wavell, *Allenby*, 195.
11. C. Searle, 'Bilharziasis and Malaria during the Palestine Campaign,' *Journal of the Royal Army Medical Corps* 34 (1920): 15–34; Yekutiel, 'Masterman, Muehlens and Malaria.'
12. Luce, 'War Experiences,' 465.

13. Hill, *Chauvel of the Light Horse*, 139.
14. Wavell, *Allenby*, 255–56.
15. Luce, 'War Experiences,' 530.
16. Gullett, *Australian Imperial Force*, 642, 679.
17. E.P. Sewell and A.S.M. Macgregor, 'An Anti-malaria Campaign in Palestine, *Journal of the Royal Army Medical Corps* 34 (1920): 85–100; 204–18.
18. Acting Sgt. James Eneas Scott, 2nd London Sanitary Company, RAMC, IWM Document no. 79/1/1.
19. Francis D. Boyd, 'Experiences of a Consulting Physician on Duty on the Palestine Lines of Communications,' *Edinburgh Medical Journal* 22 (1919): 276–87.
20. Searle, 'Bilharziasis and Malaria.'
21. Luce, 'War Experiences,' 529–30. This dispute is well reflected in the following literature: Searle, 'Bilharziasis and Malaria'; Boyd, 'Experiences of a Consulting Physician'; G.T. Rawnsley, R.A. Cunningham, and J. Warnock, 'The Prophylaxis of Malaria,' *Journal of the Royal Army Medical Corps* 38 (1922): 400–401.
22. Manson-Bahr, 'Experiences in Malaria'; Boyd, 'Experiences of a Consulting Physician.'
23. Sewell and Macgregor, 'An Anti-malaria Campaign in Palestine.'
24. W. Evans, 'Anti-malarial Work with the Australian Mounted Division in Palestine. *Medical Journal of Australia* (1919) part II: 526–29.
25. Searle, 'Bilharziasis and Malaria.'
26. Powles, *New Zealanders*, 261.
27. Luce, 'War Experiences,' 529–30. Surgeon-General Luce cited from General Viscount Wolsley's *Soldier's Pocket-Book*, 5th ed. (London: MacMillan, 1886), 110. Though the citation is correct, its interpretation by Luce is quite misleading. Wolsley's ideas should be interpreted in the context of his time, when they were written. He referred to 'sanitation' as it was defined and understood at that time, when the new 'germ theory' had not yet been accepted by many physicians. Thus, when Luce made the comparison between the two Generals, he meant well; however, he ignored the historical context.
28. Sewell and Macgregor, 'An Anti-malaria Campaign in Palestine.'
29. Gen. Allenby to Gen. Wilson, 5 June 1918, Wilson Papers, IWM, HHW2/33A/4.
30. Gray, *Red Dust*, 141.
31. Lovegrove, *Not Least in the Crusade*, 45–46.

CHAPTER EIGHT

1. Order of Battle of the EEF, 18 September 1918, in Falls, *Military Operations [...] from June 1917 to the End of the War*, 2:666–73. Each Indian Infantry Divisions had five field ambulances. They usually consisted of 5 sections: 2 British and 3 Indian. There were cases in which these field ambulances included only 4 sections: 2 British and 2 Indian. As these units included both British and Indian sections, they were called 'Combined Field Ambulances.' An Indian Cavalry Division also included 5 Combined Field Ambulances, each consisting of 5 sections: 2 British and 3 Indian. Thus an Indian Division usually included 25 field ambulance sections. See BGGS EEF HQ document describing EEF medical units, 11 Sept. 1918, PRO WO 95/4371.
2. Donald Macdonald, *Surgeons Twoe and Barber: Being some Account of the Life and Work of the Indian Medical Service (1600–1947)* (London: Heinemann, 1950), 174. The hospitals were Nos. 39, 41, 44, 50, 51, and 54 Indian General Hospitals. While a British General Hospital included 520 beds and 358 personnel, the Indian General Hospital had 500 beds and 270

personnel. An Egyptian Detention Hospital included 180 beds, while an Egyptian Stationary Hospital had either 600 or 1,000 beds. See PRO WO 95/4371 (previous note).

3. Secret 0 1/138/395: 'Future Operations in Palestine,' 26 Dec. 1917, PRO WO 106/728.
4. Falls, *Military Operations [...] from June 1917 to the End of the War*, 1:310–11.
5. Wavell, *Palestine Campaigns*, 192–99; Cyril Falls, *Armageddon, 1918* (Annapolis, MD: Nautical & Aviation Pub. Co. of America, 1979), 35–49.
6. Barrett, 'The Halford Oration.'
7. Training of the new divisions included the issue of 'medical arrangements', as reflected by the scheme for tactical exercise for the 5th Cavalry Division, 14 Sept. 1918, PRO WO 95/4517.
8. Abraham, *Surgeon's Journey*, 228–29.
9. EEF GHQ, Preliminary order for location of hospitals during the offensive, August 1918, PRO WO 95/4749.
10. Butler, *Official History*, 717 n. 5.
11. Scheme for tactical exercise for the 5th Cavalry Division (n. 7 abve), PRO WO 95/4517; document concerning training of the 7 Indian Division, WO 95/4707.
12. 'DDMS Desert Mounted Corps Medical Services Operation Order No. 5,' 14 Sept. 1918, in Butler, *Official History*, Appendix 4, 821–24.
13. Ibid., 717. The only details concerning this experimental drop could be found in the biography of General Chauvel: 'At the request of Colonel Downes, DDMS of the Desert Corps, Ross Smith had dropped tyre tubes filled with food from 2000 feet on 17 September. Downes noted in his diary that the experiment was a success." See Hill, *Chauvel of the Light Horse*, 165, n. One may easily relate these preparations to the previous experience of medical supply by airplanes, initiated by Colonel R.M. Downes, during the second raid into Transjordan. It might also be recalled that Ross Smith, an Australian pilot who served in Palestine, had previously served as a gunner in the Light Horse during the Dardanelles Campaign. Only after that did he become a pilot. This could explain his relations and enthusiastic cooperation with Colonel Downes.
14. Medical arrangements for the 10th Division, written by the ADMS, Colonel G.T.K. Maurice, PRO WO 95/4571; Medical arrangements for the 53th Division, written by the ADMS, Colonel E.J.R Evatt, PRO WO 95/4618.
15. Dalbiac, *History of the 60th Division*, 221.
16. Abraham, *Surgeon's Journey*, 228–29, 231. Dr Abraham also wrote the following about Surgeon General Swan in the Official Medical History of the War: 'Major-General Swan, as he then was, had by this time organized the medical services during the difficult period of reconstructing the medical units for British and Indians and for the coming final operations. After his departure these final medical preparations, under his administration, underwent no alteration, and proved remarkably efficient.' See Macpherson, *Medical Services: General History*, 3:464.
17. A vast literature has been published dealing with the issue of 'shell shock' during the Great War. Most of the reports originated from the Western Front. Several publications might be quite enlightening: Carl May, 'Lord Moran's Memoir: Shell-shock and the Pathology of Fear,' *Journal of the Royal Society of Medicine* 91 (1998): 95–100; P.S. Ellis, 'The Origin of the War Neuroses, parts I & II,' ibid., 70 (1984): 168–77; 71 (1985): 32–44; W.A. Turner, 'Neuroses and Psychoses of War,' *Journal of the Royal Army Medical Corps* 31 (1918): 399–413. About how the psychological impact of war was understood or misunderstood at that time, see Whitehead, *Doctors in the Great War*, 168; Ben Shepherd, *A War of Nerves* (Cambridge, MA: Harvard University Press, 2001).
18. Diary of the 53th Division HQ, 20 Sept. 1918, PRO WO 95/4617.

19. Falls, *Military Operations [...] from June 1917 to the End of the War*, 2:509.
20. Ibid., 2:510.
21. Abraham, *Surgeon's Journey*, 233.
22. Hector Dinning, *Nile to Aleppo: With the Light-Horse in the Middle-East* (London: G. Allen & Unwin, 1920), 210–11.
23. Macpherson, *Medical Services: General History*, 3:470.
24. Gen. Allenby to his wife, 21 Sept. 1918, LHMCA, Allenby Papers, 1/9.
25. Luce, 'War Experiences,' 582; EEF HQ, Sept. 1918, PRO WO 95/4371.
26. Butler, *Official History*, 723.
27. Hughes, *Allenby and British Strategy*, 100.
28. Falls, *Military Operations [...] from June 1917 to the End of the War*, Appendix 27, 2:723.
29. Gullett, *Australian Imperial Force*, 562.
30. General Allenby's letter to the troops, 26 Sept. 1918; LHMCA, Allenby Papers, Document No. 800/2/5/5.
31. Falls, *Military Operations [...] from June 1917 to the End of the War*, 2:583. For this unusual and terrible event and the attempts to justify it by a previous massacre committed by the Turks, see also Barrow, *Fire of Life*:

    'There are statements in the same book [Robert Graves, *With Lawrence and the Arabs*] which are also to be found in Lawrence's own book, Revolt in the Desert that are not in accordance with actual facts or are entirely suppostitious' (p. 209).

    'Turks, some dead and some dying, lay about the railway station or sat propped against the houses. Those still living gazed at us with eyes that begged for a little of the mercy which it was hopeless for them to ask of the Arabs [...]. In all this there was nothing that is uncommon in war. But a revolting scene was being enacted at the moment when we entered, far exceeding in its savagery anything that has been known in the conflicts between nations during the past 120 years and happily rare even in earlier times

    A long ambulance train full of sick and wounded Turks was drawn up in the station. In the cab of the engine was the dead driver and a mortally wounded fireman. The Arab soldiers were going through the train, tearing off the clothing of the groaning and stricken Turks, regardless of gaping wounds and broken limbs, and cutting their victims throats. The atrocities which the Turks are said to have inflicted on the Arab people gave cause for vengeance. But it was a sight that no average civilized human being could bear unmoved. I asked Lawrence to remove the Arabs. He said he couldn't "as it was their idea of war." I replied "It is not our idea of war, and if you can't remove them, I will." He said "If you attempt to do that I shall take no responsibility as to what happens." I answered "That's all right; I will take the responsibility," and at once gave orders for our men to clear the station. This was done and nothing untoward happened. All the Arabs were turned off the train and it was picqueted by our sentries' (p. 211).

    See also Lawrence, *Revolt in the Desert*, 307–11; Preston, *Desert Mounted Corps*, 264–65.

CHAPTER NINE

1. Lawrence, *Seven Pillars of Wisdom*, Chapter CXX, 646.
2. Butler, *Official History*, 734–35; Hughes, *Allenby and British Strategy*, 101.
3. The diary of the ADMS, the Australian Mounted Division, PRO WO 95/4553; T.E. Lawrence, though describing the situation at the hospital in a very similar way, gives a very different account of how the problem had been handled and solved. See Lawrence, *Seven Pillars of Wisdom*, Chapter CXXI, 650–52.

4. The English Hospital had been functioning undisturbed until the British Cavalry stormed Nazareth in September. When the Turkish units, including General Liman von Sanders' GHQ, retreated to Damascus, they took with them the nurses from the hospital.
5. Hughes, *Allenby and British Strategy*, 101; Macpherson, *Medical Services: General History*, 3:478–79.
6. There were no real medical units, nor a medical infrastructure, in the Arab army. However, from the outset of British military involvement in the Arab Revolt, Medical Officers had been sent from Cairo, on a personal basis, to provide medical assistance when needed. The first doctor to join the Arab Army was Captain (later Major) W.E. Marshall, RAMC, who came to the Hedjaz already in 1916, with Lt-Colonel Stuart Newcombe. Dr Marshall did his best to treat casualties and sick troops. In Akaba he even established a medical facility in a hut. For Marshall and his efforts, see Lawrence, *Revolt in the Desert*, 226, 228, 261, 264, 287, 311, 329, 349, and more. Lawrence wrote: '[At Azrak, during the advance to Damascus] Marshall at the temporary hospital. He had all our badly-wounded in his quiet care; but they were fewer than he had expected, so he was able to spare me a stretcher for my bed' (ibid., 390). Marshall is also mentioned by Lawrence in *Seven Pillars of Wisdom*, Chapter CVII. Urgent medical support was sent from Cairo to Akaba when the Arabs faced an outbreak of cholera there (see Chapter 2 above).
7. Dr Ramsey was, most probably, one of the few doctors who joined the Arab army during the last phase of the war. According to one source, he was 'acting as Principal MO of the Sherifian army' (Butler, *Official History*, 734).
8. Abraham, *Surgeon's Journey*, 236.
9. The diary of the ADMS, the Australian Mounted Division, PRO WO 95/4553; Macpherson, *Medical Services: General History*, 3:478; Abraham, *Surgeon's Journey*, 235–36.
10. Butler, *Official History*, 733.
11. Macpherson, *Medical Services: General History*, 3:479.
12. Ibid., 3:478.
13. Gullett, *Australian Imperial Force*, 777.
14. Memoir of Major R.H. Wilson, Berkshire Yeomanry, the 5th Mounted Brigade, IWM 82/25/1, 66.
15. For the 'Ludendorff Offensive' see Chapter 6 above.
16. Much has been written concerning Spanish Flue. Most of the works deal with the etiology and epidemiology of the disease in the US and in Europe. There is no real epidemiologic data base concerning the disease in the Middle East. A good general review of Spanish Flue may be found in John M. Barry, *The Great Influenza: The Epic Story of the Deadliest Plague in History* (London: Penguin Books, 2004).
17. It is interesting to note that cases of Spanish Flue were treated in various places around the world with quinine injections, as it was assumed that it might enhance the activity of the immune system. See Barry, *The Great Influenza*, 353, 403.
18. Macpherson, *Medical Services: General History*, 3:476–79.
19. Butler, *Official History*, 747–51.
20. Salaman, *Palestine Reclaimed*, 94–95. Dr. Salaman was confusing two different Jewish medical organizations. The Haddasah Medical Organization was founded in the US in 1912 with the goal of promoting the health of the Jewish population in Palestine. The first two nurses arrived in Jerusalem in 1913 but were compelled to leave Palestine during the war. In 1916, the Hadassah Organization purchased the Rothschild Hospital in Jerusalem but only in November 1918 could it actually be opened. However, in June 1918, a delegation of the American Zionist Medical Unit (AZMU) arrived in Jerusalem. It included doctors, specializing in most branches of medicine, and nurses. This group would in a few months

open the Hadassah hospital in Jerusalem but in the meantime tried to help the local population by supplying health services. Dr Salaman was referring to this group – AZMU – which at the time of the great offensive was operating in Jerusalem.

21. Abraham, *Surgeon's Journey*, 235–36.
22. 'The Desert Mounted Corps rode through the Turkish line near Jaffa with a force of 27,500 men. At the end of the campaign they had lost 633 killed and wounded and 11,300 men from malaria and some influenza. Chaytor's Force, which consisted of 13,000 men, lost during the final offensive 139 soldiers on the battlefield and 8,352 to malaria' (Barrett, 'The Halford Oration').
23. Falls, *Armageddon*, 99.
24. Pellagra was first described in Spain in 1762. It was first reported in Egypt in 1847 by Prumner. There were several publications concerning the cases of the disease among the Turkish prisoners of war: A.D. Bigland, 'Oedema as a Symptom in So-called Food-deficiency Disease,', *Lancet* (1920) part I: 243–47; idem, 'The Pellagra Outbreak in Egypt,' ibid.: 947–53, 998–1003; J.I. Enright, 'War Eedema in Turkish Prisoners of War,' ibid.: 314–16; H.M. Woodcock, 'Helminthic Infections in Relation to Pellagra,' ibid.: 1193–95.
25. LHMCA, Allenby Papers, 6/8.
26. Allenby to Wilson, 22 Oct. 1918, IWM, Wilson Papers, HHW2/33a/27; cited as Letter No. 185 in *Allenby in Palestine*, p. 210.
27. 'The Pellagra Report,' WIHM, Document No. RAMC 567 It might be very interesting to note that the 'Pellagra Committee' – as well as other British investigators at the time – was not aware of the work done by Goldberger and his co-workers in the United States. The etiology of Pellagra was conclusively discovered by Goldberger only in September 1927 ('Pellagra, Its Nature and Prevention,' *Public Health Reports* 42, no. 35 [2 Sept. 1927]: 2193–2200. The following was written in a volume of the General History of the Medical Services published in 1922: 'There is no special bibliography which deals with pellagra during the war, but a very extensive bibliography is published in a work on Pellagra by Dr. A.F. Harris, of Atlanta, in 1919', see *Medical Services: Diseases of the War*, ed. William G. Macpherson [et al.], 2 vols., History of the Great War, Based on Official Documents (London: HMSO, 1922), 1:470–84. Robert McCarrison, at the time an authority on deficiency diseases, wrote after the war:'Goldberger and his colleagues have established the fact that a close relationship exists between food deficiency and Pellagra. They consider that the deficiency may be one of suitable protein, of vitamins, of mineral salts, or more probably of a combination of two or more of these. The work of the Committee of Inquiry, regarding the prevalence of Pellagra among Turkish prisoners of war in Egypt, has also emphasized the connexion between Pellagra and defective protein supply to the body tissues. This committee considered that the defective protein supply may be due either to inadequate intake of protein of good biological value or to the malassimilation of such protein.' Robert McCarrisson, *Studies in Deficiency Disease* (London: Henry Frowde and Hodder and Stoughton, 1921), 228.
28. 'Medicine in the War – Second Notice,' *British Medical Journal* (1922) part II: 761–62. The DMS, Colonel Richard Luce, wrote to Lt-Colonel P.S. Lelean: 'I have read through the report on the Pellagra work. It is a monumental work and a model of clear reasoning. I am sending a copy on to "A" with my remarks and I propose to send a copy to the Director General with a request to have it published. [...] I think you have made out a very strong case for the Biological Proteins. There certainly seems absolutely no evidence in any other direction. I feel that the Commission has done great good in clearing away possible risk of post-war cavillings and thank you both for the splendid way in which you have tackled it.' Luce to Lelean, 6 Jan. 1919, Letter No. 5413s, WIHM, RAMC 567.
29. Despatch of General Allenby to the CIGS, 31 Oct. 1918. Cited in *A Brief Record of the*

Advance of the Egyptian Expeditionary Force under the Command of General Sir Edmund H.H. Allenby, July 1917 to October 1918, 2d ed. (London: HMSO, 1919), 36.

EPILOGUE

1. Powles, *New Zealanders*, 264–67.
2. 'Obituary: Sir Richard Luce, K.C.M.G., C.B., F.R.C.S.,' *British Medical Journal* (1952) part I: 493–94, 662.
3. Hill, *Chauvel of the Light Horse*, 67.
4. Abraham, *Surgeon's Journey*, 244–45.

INDEX

Basic Anglicised spelling without diacritical marks has been used in the transliteration of Arabic and Hebrew names. It follows the usage in the Official Histories, even if this deviates at times from accepted spellings today.

The index does not include references to General Edmund H.H. Allenby, the major protagonist of this book.

APPENDIX

DESERT MOUNTED CORPS

Australian Mounted Division.
3rd, 4th, 5th Australian light Horse Brigades.
Australian & New Zealand (ANZAC) Mounted Division.
1st, 2nd Australian Light Horse Brigades; New Zealand Mounted Rifles Brigade.
Yeomanry Mounted Division
6th, 8th, 22nd Mounted Brigades.
7th Mounted Brigade
Imperial Camel Corps Brigade

XX CORPS

53rd (Welsh) Division
158th, 159th, 160th Brigades.
60th (London) Division
179th, 180th, 181st Brigades.
74th Division
229th, 230th, 231st Brigades.
10th (Irish) Division
29th, 30th, 31st Brigades.

XXI CORPS

52nd (Lowland) Division.
  155th, 156th, 157th Brigades.
54th (East Anglian) Division.
  161st, 162nd, 163th Brigades.
75th Division.
  232nd, 233rd, 234th Brigades.

EGYPTIAN EXPEDITIONARY FORCE, SEPTEMBER 1918

DESERT MOUNTED CORPS

4th Cavalry Division.
  10th, 11th, 12th Cavalry Brigades.
5th Cavalry Division.
  13th, 14th, 15th cavalry brigades.
Australian Mounted Division.
  3rd, 4th, 5th Australian Light Horse Brigades.

XX CORPS

10th Division
  29th, 30th, 31st Brigades.
53rd Division
  158th, 159th, 160th Brigades.

XXI CORPS

3rd (Lahore) Division.
  7th, 8th, 9th Brigades.
7th (Meerut) Division.
  19th, 21st, 28th Brigades.
54th Division.
  161st, 162nd, 163rd Brigades.

60th Division.
179th, 180th, 181st Brigades.
75th Division.
232nd, 233rd, 234th Brigades.
Detachement Francais de Palestine et Syrie.

CHAYTOR'S FORCE

Australian & New Zealand (ANZAC) Mounted Division.
1st, 2nd Australian Light Horse Brigades, New Zealand Mounted Rifles Brigade.
20th Indian Brigade.

ARMY MEDICAL SERVICES

DIVISIONAL FIELD AMBULANCES

ANZAC Mounted Division.
1st, 2nd, Light Horse, and New Zealand Mounted Brigade Field Ambulances.
Australian Mounted Division.
3rd, 4th, 5th Light Horse Field Ambulances.
3rd (Lahore) Division.
110th,111th, 112th, Indian Combined Field Ambulances.
7th (Meerut) Division.
128th, 129th, 130th Indian Combined Field Ambulances.
4th Cavalry Division.
10th, 11th,12th Cavalry Brigade Combined Field Ambulances.
5th Cavalry Division.
13th, 14th, 15th Cavalry Brigade Combined Field Ambulances.
10th Division.
Until Spring 1918 : 30th, 31st, 32nd Field Ambulances.
From Spring 1918 : 154th, 165th, 166th Indian Combined Field Ambulances.

52nd Division.

1/1st, 1/2nd, 1/3rd Lowland Field Ambulances.

53rd Division.

Until Spring 1918 : 1/1st, 1/2nd, 1/3rd Welsh Field Ambulances.

From Spring 1918 : 1/1st Welsh Field Ambulance, 113th, 170th, 171st Indian Combined Field Ambulances.

54th Division.

2/1st, 1/2nd, 1/3rd East Anglian Field Ambulances.

60th Division.

Until Spring 1918 : 2/4th, 2/5th, 2/6th London Field Ambulances.

From Spring 1918 : 121st, 160th,179th Indian Combined Field Ambulances.

74th Division.

229th, 230th, 231st Field Ambulances.

75th Division.

Until Spring 1918 : 145th, 146th, 147th Field Ambulances.

From Spring 1918 : 123rd, 127th, 163rd Indian Combined Field Ambulances.

Palestine Lines of Communication.

Scottish Horse Field Ambulance.

CASUALTY CLEARING STATIONS AND CLEARING HOSPITALS

Palestine Lines of Communication.

26th, 35th, 66th, 74th, 76th Casualty Clearing Stations (CCS).

Until Spring 1918 : 65th, 75th, 77th Casualty Clearing Stations.

From Spring 1918 : 32nd, 33rd, 34th Combined Clearing Hospitals.

15th Combined Clearing Hospital.

24th Indian Clearing Hospital.

31st Indian Clearing Hospital.

Stationary Hospitals.

Palestine Lines of Communication.

24th, 26th, 36th, 43rd, 44th, 45th, 47th, 48th Stationary Hospitals.

No. 2 Australian Stationary Hopital.

137th Indian Stationary Hospital.

Hospital Trains and Barges.

Nos. 40, 44, 45, 46, 47, 48, 50, 51, 56.

Hospital Barge "Niagra"

Sanitary sections, laboratories, medical store depots.

HOSPITALS AND CONVALESCENT DEPOTS

Palestine Lines of Communication.

69th, 78th General Hospitals.

No. 14 Australian General Hospital.

Nos. 5, 30, 32, 39, 41, 44, 50, 54 Indian General Hospitals.

Nos. 3,4,5 Prisoners of Ear Hospitals.

Nos. 1,2,3,4 Egyptian Stationary Hospitals.

Nos. 1,3,4,5,6,7,8,9,10,11,12 Egyptian detention Hospitals.

Egypt.

27th, 31st, 71st General Hospitals.

31st, 45th Indian general Hospitals, Citadel Hospital, Nasrieh Hospital.

No 13 Egyptian Detention Hospital

Nos. 1,2,6,7,8,9 Prisoners of War Hospitals.

Hospitals at Alexandria District.

Convalescent Depots.